Boundary Features Classifying Chronic Liver Disease

ndar Features Classifying Chronic Liver
sease

st Edition January 2024

ritten by Daniel V

TABLE OF CONTENTS

LIST OF TABLES

LIST OF FIGURES

LIST OF SYMBOLS AND ABBREVIATIONS

4NNBPA	-	4-Class Neural Network Back Propagation Model
5MPNN	-	5-Multilayer Perceptron Neural Network
A	-	Adaboost
ACC	-	Accuracy
ALT	-	Alanine Transaminase
AFP	-	Alpha-Fetoprotein
ADT	-	Alternating Decision Tree
ANN	-	Artificial Neural Network
AST	-	Aspartate Aminotransferase
BPN	-	Back Propagation Network
BSCWPT	-	Back Scan Converted Wavelet Packet Transform
B	-	Bayes
BWSTF	-	Biorthogonal Wavelet Based Statistical Texture Feature
BWT	-	Biorthogonal Wavelet Transform
CFFBPN	-	Cascade Feed Forward Back Propagation Network
CH	-	Chronic Hepatic
CLD	-	Chronic Liver disease
C	-	Cirrhosis
CS	-	Classification Step
CLR 1	-	Classifier 1
CLR 2	-	Classifier 2
CLR 3	-	Classifier 3
CBC	-	Clinical Based Classifier
CA	-	Clustering Algorithm

CAC	_	Color Auto Correlation
CH	_	Color Histogram
CM	_	Color Moment
CC	_	Compensated Cirrhosis
CT	_	Computed Tomography
CCCM	_	Contour Coefficient Co-occurrence Matrices
CCFOS	_	Contour Coefficient First Order Statistics
CLAHE	_	Contrast Limited Adaptive Histogram Equalization
CNN	_	Convolutional Neural Network
CM	_	Co-occurrence Matrix
DM	_	Data Mining
DT	_	Decision Tree
DC	_	Decompensated Cirrhosis
DL	_	Deep Learning
DIF	_	Despeckle Image Filter
DR	_	Detection Rate
Σ_i	_	Diagonal Covariance Matrix
DWT	_	Discrete Wavelet Transform
DBFCC	_	Discriminant Boundary Features based Clinical Classifiers
ELM-HHOG	_	Ensemble Learning Machine-Hough Histogram Oriented Gradient
ELM-RFE	_	Extreme Learning Machine-Recursive Features Elimination
FDCT	_	Fast Discrete Curvelet Transform
FFNN	_	Feed Forward Neural Network
FOS	_	First Order Statistics
FFVBWT	_	Fractal Feature Vector Based Wavelet Transform

FDTA	-	Fractional Dimensional Textural Analysis
FL	-	Fuzzy Logic
gGT	-	Gamma Glutamyl Transpeptidase
GMM	-	Gaussian Mixture Model
GA	-	Genetic Algorithm
GLCM	-	Gray Level Co-occurrence Matrices
GLDM	-	Gray Level Difference Matrix
GLDS	-	Gray Level Difference Statistics
GLFOS	-	Gray Level First Order Statistics
GLRLM	-	Gray Level Run Length Matrix
RUNL	-	Gray Level Run Length Statistics
HBV	-	Hepatitis B Virus
HCV	-	Hepatitis C Virus
HMM	-	Hidden Markov Model
H	-	Hierarchical
HFF	-	Hierarchical Feature of Fuzzy
HOS	-	Higher Order Statistics
HOG	-	Histogram Oriented Gradient
HHOG	-	Hough Histogram Oriented Gradient
HFOS	-	Hybrid First Order Statistics
IDT	-	Intensity Difference Technique
INR	-	International Normalized Ratio
IDM	-	Inverse Difference Moment
KM	-	K-mean
KNN	-	K Nearest Neighbor
LVQ	-	Learning Vector Quantization
LOOCV	-	Leave One Out Cross Validation
LIBSVM	-	Library Support Vector Machine

LPM	-	Liver Probability Map
LDH	-	Locate Dehydrogenase
ML	-	Machine Learning
MLA	-	Machine Learning Algorithm
MR-E	-	Magnetic Resonance Elastrography
MRI	-	Magnetic Resonance Imaging
MR-S	-	Magnetic Resonance Spectrography
MSE	-	Mean Square Error
MPSO	-	Modified Particle Swarm Optimization
α	-	Moore Penrose Inverse Matrix
MA	-	Morphological Algorithm
MREG	-	Multi Linear Regression
MSVM	-	Multi Support Vector Machine
NN	-	Neural Networks
NFLD	-	Non-alcoholic Fatty Liver Disease
NSWT	-	Non Separable Wavelet Transform
N	-	Normal
μ_i	-	Normal Vector
OA	-	Optimization Algorithm
OROI	-	Optimum Region Of Interest
OA	-	Overall Accuracy
PSO	-	Particle Swarm Optimization
P	-	Pathologic
PSNR	-	Peak Signal to Noise Ratio
PCA	-	Principle Component Analysis
PNN	-	Probabilistic Neural Network
PT	-	Processing Time
RBF	-	Radial Bias Function

RF	-	Random Forest
RGB	-	Red Green Blue
ROC	-	Region Of Classifier
ROI	-	Region Of Interest
RFSFSWM	-	Releif Filter Sequential Forward Selection Wrapper Method
w_i	-	Scalar Weight
SIFT	-	Scale Invariant Feature Transform
SN	-	Sensitivity
SBS	-	Sequential Backward Selection
SFFS	-	Sequential Forward Floating Search
SFS	-	Sequential Forward Selection
SGLDM	-	Spatial Gray Level Dependence Matrices
SP	-	Specificity
SIF	-	Speckle Image Filter
SR	-	Stepwise Regression
SVM	-	Support Vector Machine
TA	-	Topological Analysis
US	-	Ultrasound
ULM-HE	-	Unsupervised Learning Machine-Histogram Equalization
WPT	-	Wavelet Packet transform
WOASA	-	Whale Optimization Algorithm Stimulated Annealing
J	-	Youden's Index

CHAPTER 1

INTRODUCTION TO CHRONIC LIVER DISEASE

Healthy life is medicine free life. All human organs need to b healthy and work correctly. Liver is the largest internal organ. It lies und the right ribs. The liver weights about 3 pounds. It has an extraordina property of self-regeneration to its original size and shape.

The liver shape is chock like structure and shielded over wi ribcage. It is built up of hepatic cells which differ from millions primary metabolic cells. It removes waste from the body, such as toxins ar medicines, making bile to help digest food, storing sugar that the body use for energy and making new proteins.

Metabolism, removing toxic substances, excretion of bile in intestine, and generation of the protein are the primary function of th liver. Excretion is used to increase the digestion process. Generation protein is used to prevent clotting of blood.

Repeated series of inflammation (fibrosis), necrosis, ar hepatocellular regeneration lead to the growth of liver cirrhosis. There is great difference between the individuals who are affected by Hepatitis. differs for every individual. Most of the research reports provide som sufficient evidence that the disease is due to multiple factors like genetic host immunological system, long term viral effects, environmental factors ar so on.

Liver is present for both vertebrates and other animals. It is the largest gland in the human body. Prevention of liver damage is very important because of its very important functions like decomposition of red blood cells, plasma protein synthesis and detoxification and glycogen storage. So liver damage has to be detected earlier.

Liver diseases can be classified into two main classes according to the level of dispersion of the diseases. They have Spread Liver Diseases and Vital Liver Diseases. The classification does not indicate that the first category is a later stage of the second or that it is more serious. They should be treated in totally different possible ways. Fatty liver is the increase of fat in the liver cells. Fat assembles in the liver with a number of conditions. The most general factor is obesity. Fatty liver is also related to diabetes, triglycerides and the use of alcohol.

Chronic Hepatitis is a syndrome of chronic inflammation of liver disease classified by continuing hepatocytic damage related with abnormal conditions. Excess alcohol ingestion is one of the major causes of chronic liver disease. Classically, alcoholic liver damage includes three major forms: 1. fatty liver, 2. chronic hepatitis and 3. cirrhosis. The amount and time duration of alcohol intake are the most important risk factors involved in the development of the chronic liver disease. Chronic liver disease may lead to chronic hepatitis.

Examination of patients with liver disease should be directed at 1. Establishing the aetiologic diagnosis, 2. Estimating seriousness of the disease and 3. Establishing the different stages of disease. Diagnosis should concentrate on the finding of a specific class of the disease.

Grading refers to evaluating the seriousness or activity of disease such as active or inactive, small or medium or severe. Staging refers to

calculating the place in the course of the history of the disease, wheth
critical or chronic, early or late, precirrhosis, cirrhosis or end-stage.

1.1 CHRONIC LIVER DISEASE

CLD is a persistent disease that may increase the morbidity a
temporality rate in advanced countries and is commonly caused by vir
hepatitis and long term alcohol usage. The beginning stages of CLD a
generally asymptomatic such as hepatitis. Hepatitis is a very usual disease th
causes the inflammation of the liver. Liver inflammation can be caus
because of some agent's like parasites virus, alcohol and other chemicals.

1.1.1 Symptoms of Chronic Liver Disease

Chronic Liver Disease includes fluid accumulation in the bel
(ascites), vomiting blood, bleeding in the blood vessels in the food pi
(esophagus), gallstones, itching, yellowing of the skin and eyes (jaundice
kidney failure, muscle loss and loss of appetite.

1.1.2 Roots of Chronic Liver Disease

The most useful roots of Chronic Liver Disease are Hepatitis a
other viruses. The major factors are Long term alcohol abuse a
Nonalcoholic fatty liver disease. Nonalcoholic fatty liver disease happe
from metabolic syndrome. Nonalcoholic fatty liver disease (NFLD) is caus
by obesity, high cholesterol, triglycerides and high blood pressure.

1.1.3 Treatment for Chronic Liver Disease

Chronic liver disease is a progressive liver disease that happe
over time. The damage to liver can sometimes reverse or improve if th
proper treatment is done, by treating a viral infection or by not drinkir

alcohol. The objective of treatment is to slow down the buildup of scar tissue and prevent or treat other health problems.

In many cases, treatment delays or stops any more liver damage. Chronic Liver Disease is treated to delay worsening of the liver disease. Treatment includes eating a healthy diet, low in sodium, not using alcohol or illegal drugs and managing any health problems because of chronic liver disease.

1.2 STAGES OF CHRONIC LIVER DISEASE

Due to alcoholism, viral infections, metabolic disorders, therapeutic agents and changed immunity have grown to the development of CLD. The disease can be split into 3 stages.

1.2.1 Chronic Hepatitis

The first stage is the chronic hepatitis. Chronic hepatitis is caused due to the chronic inflammation of liver (Carey (2010), Leroy *et al.* (2007)).

1.2.2 Compensated Cirrhosis

The second stage is compensated cirrhosis. The decay of cells, inflammation and fibrous deepening of the tissue give rise to compensated cirrhosis. Compensated cirrhosis arises from the serious condition of chronic hepatic disease which is asymptomatic and hence remains unknown. (Kasper *et al.* (2015)).

1.2.3 Decompensated Cirrhosis

The third stage is decompensated cirrhosis. Decompensate cirrhosis is the advanced stage with severe symptoms, which often ends death. The symptoms include ascites, jaundice, gastro- intestinal bleedin thrombocytopenia and hepatic encephalopathy. The end-stage of this disea is death or Hepatocellular carcinoma (Kasper *et al.* (2015)).

1.3 LIVER BIOPSY

Liver biopsy is the reference standard method for the classificatic and staging of chronic liver diseases. Invasive and noninvasive methods a used to estimate the pathogenicity of the liver. To establish that the liver diseased, so many investigations are done such as physical examinatio laboratory tests, imaging or scanning the abdomen area and performing Liv Biopsy.

1.3.1 Invasive Method

The analysis is done by the invasive method to assess a liv biopsy. The results allow some kind of hurdles such as pain after liv biopsy. The problems are pneumo- thorax, bleeding, puncture of th biliary tree and rarely death due to over bleeding. Liver biopsy is avoide in the first stage. For the above circumstances noninvasive methods a used as a secondary for liver biopsy.

1.3.2 Noninvasive Method

Particularly, the fibro test, fibro meter, transient elastography (U based technology), hepascore and aspartate platelet ratio index are th noninvasive methods for determining the liver conditio (Gaiani et al. (1997), Schuppan Detlef & Nezam H Afdhal (2008))

1.3.2.1 Fibro Test

Fibro test is used to estimate the fibrosis and inflammatory function of the liver as shown in figure 1.1. Six serum markers α2-macroglobulin, haptoglobulin, bilirubin, gamma Glutamyl trans peptidase, Apo lipoprotein and alanine transferase are the tests included in the fibro test. Fibro test shows some inaccurate results; hence it is not preferred in most of the hospitals. Fibro test uses the results of six blood serum tests to generate a value that is mapped with the level of liver damage (Poynard *et al.* (2007)). Hence, some typical kinds of classification method can be used in earlier stage detection by identifying the health conditions with some pathologic conditions.

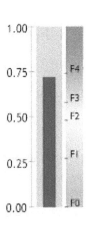

Figure 1.1 Fibro Test

1.3.2.2 Fibro Meter

Fibro meter is used to measure liver disease as shown in figure 1.2. The test includes α2-macroglobulin, prothrombin time, platelets and hyaluronate. It gives an accurate result for chronic viral hepatitis. Fibro meter is a blood test used to calculate the liver fibrosis (Cales *et al.* (2008)).

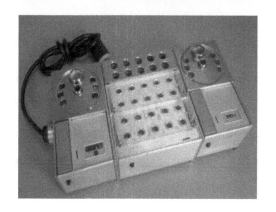

Figure 1.2 Fibro Meter

1.3.2.3   Transient Elastography

Another form of transient elastography is a fibro scan as show
in figure 1.3. It works by the principle of shear wave (Kim *et al.* (2013)
By using an ultrasound probe, a shear wave is sent through the liver. She
wave velocity is observed to the liver stiffness. It generates the output
kilopascals. The ultrasound transducer is the Fibro meter.

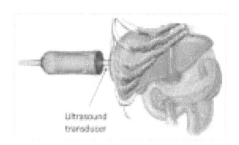

Figure 1.3 Ultrasound Transducer

1.3.2.4   Hepascore

HE employs gamma glutamyl transpeptidase, hyaluronic acid, alpha
macroglobulin and bilirubin. Hepascore is another liver function test obtaine
from serum analytes capable of accurately predicting the extent of liver fibros
in patients with hepatitis C infection (Adams *et al.* (2005)).

1.3.2.5   Aspartate Platelet Ratio Index

Aspartate aminotransferase / platelet ratio index forecast the fibrosis and cirrhosis in hepatitis C patients. It is a non-invasive way to predict which patients have cirrhosis without imaging or biopsy (Yilmaz *et al.* (2011).

1.3.2.6   Drawbacks

When compared to the single method, combined methods give a better analysis. These methods are not a better substitute biopsy since they have some limitations with the absence of infrastructure.

1.4   DIAGONSIS OF LIVER DISEASE

Blood tests, imaging tests and Tissue analysis are used to diagnose the liver disease.

1.4.1   Physical Examination

The physical examination normally formals rather than replaces the need for other diagnostic approaches. In many patients, the physical examination is normal unless the disease is critical or severe and advanced. Physical findings in liver disease are icterus, hepatomegaly, hepatic tenderness, splenomegaly, spider angiomata, palmar erythema and excoriations.

Icterus is the best method by inspecting the sclera under natural light. In fair skin, a yellow color of the skin may be obvious. In dark skin, the mucous membranes below the tongue can demonstrate jaundice.

Hepatomegaly is not reliable for liver disease, because of the variability of the size and shape of the liver and the physical impediments to evaluate the liver size by percussion. The most reliable physical finding determining the liver is hepatic tenderness.

Spiral angiomata and palmar erythema occur in both critical and chronic liver disease and especially a person with cirrhosis. But they can occur in normal person and are frequently present at the time of pregnancy. Spider angiomata occur only on the arms, face and upper torso. They may be difficult to detect in dark skin.

1.4.2 Laboratory Tests

The diagnosis of liver diseases is aided by the availability of liver tests for liver damage and functions. There is no single test by which the liver can function normally. Therefore several tests are undergone in each patient and sometimes the individual test must be repeated.

1.4.3 Blood Tests

A group of blood tests called liver function tests can be used to diagnose liver disease.

1.4.4 Imaging Tests

An ultrasound, CT scan and MRI can be used to diagnose liver disease. An ultrasound, CT scan and MRI can show the liver damage.

1.4.5 Tissue Analysis

Removing a tissue sample (biopsy) from the liver may help diagnose liver disease and look for liver damage signs.

1.5   MEDICAL IMAGING

Computerized medical image processing plays an important role in various medical fields such as diagnosis, therapy planning, or monitoring. Due to the aging society and the widespread of modern imaging technologies the number of medical images to be processed increases in clinical practice.

1.5.1   Ultrasound Imaging

Medical ultrasound is one of the diagnostic imaging technique, or therapeutic application of ultrasound as shown in figure 1.4 (Joseph *et al.* (1979)). It is used to create an image of the internal body structures such as tendons, muscles, joints, blood vessels and internal organs. Its aim is often to find a source of a disease or to exclude pathology. The images of liver used in this extraction technique are collected using Ultrasonography. Ultrasound imaging uses sound waves to produce pictures of the inside of the body. It helps diagnose the causes of pain, swelling and infection in the body's internal organs, and to determine a baby in pregnant women and the brain and hips in infants. It is also used to help guide biopsies, diagnose heart conditions, and assess damage after a heart attack. Ultrasound is safe, non-invasive, and does not use ionizing radiation.

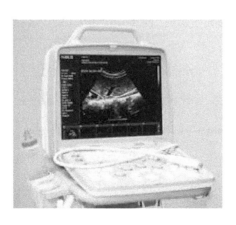

Figure 1.4 Ultrasound Imaging

1.5.2   Computed Tomography Imaging

A computerized tomography is a combination of X-ray imag taken from different angles around the body as shown in figure 1.5 (Berna et al. (2000)). It uses computer processing to create cross-sectional images the bones, blood vessels and soft tissues inside the body. A compute tomography scan image provides more detailed information than ordinary X rays do. A computed tomography scan has many applications, but it particularly well equipped to examine people who may have internal injuri from accidents or other emergency types. A computed tomography scan used to show all parts of the body. It is used to diagnose the disease or inju as well as to plan medical, surgical or radiation treatment.

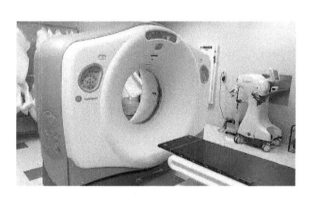

Figure 1.5 Computed Tomography Imaging

1.5.3   Magnetic Resonance Imaging

Magnetic resonance imaging is another medical imaging techniqu used in radiology to form pictures of the human body's anatomy and th physiological processes of the human body as shown in figure 1.6 (Mortele al. (2002)). Magnetic resonance imaging scanners deploy strong magnet fields, magnetic field gradients, and radio waves to produce images of th organs in the human body.

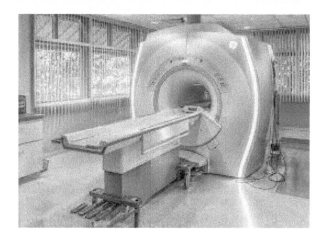

Figure 1.6 Magnetic Resonance Imaging

1.5.4 Cathode Angiography

Cathode Angiography is one of the standard methods for vascular determination of the liver before tumor reanalysis, but it is an invasive technique. However, with the current advances in computed tomography imaging or Magnetic resonance imaging technology, the non invasive determination of hepatic vessels can be performed reliably by contrast enhanced computed tomography imaging or Magnetic resonance imaging. In current scenario, Catheter Angiography is performed for therapeutic liver tumor natural formation, and to decide complex vascular study demonstrated on computed tomography imaging or Magnetic resonance imaging.

1.5.5 Positron Emission Tomography

Positron Emission Tomography is a diagnostic tool in the evaluation of metastatic liver disease. The advantages are sensitivity and the ability to cover the entire body at a single sitting. The main disadvantages include its high cost, poor availability, and poor lesion localization.

1.6 RESEARCH MOTIVATION

CLD due to the viral hepatitis and alcohol abuse have faced mar challenges like genetics, host immunological system, long term viral effec environmental factors and so on. CLD is a continuous mortal disea causing more damages to human lives. Due to CLD, there is hike in t temporality and morbidity rate in the growing countries. The condition the liver is determined using noninvasive method. The minimization liver biopsy is done by using noninvasive method as a useful diagnost tool which is the main objective. In this research, recovering, finding solution and preventing the disease from such conditions are considered as major challenging task.

1.6.1 CLD Challenges

Etiological intersect must receive observation in CLD

The patient with two or more mixed diseases should be careful identified.

Hepatic and systematic inflammation should be determined for CLD

Inflammatory evaluations have always been carried out, whi performing CLD classification, and evaluating systemic inflammation by t detecting of serum inflammatory biomarkers.

Non invasive measurements should be evolved for CLD diagnosis

Non-invasive measurements are highly applicable and easi reliable. The new evolved markers have been demonstrated to be of gre score in detecting advanced CLD with sensitivity and specificity.

Liver function and classification of different stages of CLD must be accurately calculated

It is likely to be more accurate in evaluating the disease seriousness and in predicting the diseases. Ultrasound elastography has been increasingly accepted as a non-invasive and practical approach for differentiating patients with normal and pathological conditions.

Etiological treatment is important

The etiological treatment of CLD is critical, although it is usually ignored in the decompensated stage. Patients should be initially treated with proper treatment as soon as hepatic cirrhosis virus is identified.

Maintain a sufficient blood supply in the portal vein

The liver is an organ with a dual blood supply from the portal vein and the hepatic artery. The maintenance of sufficient insertion is significant for ensuring the nourishment of the organ.

Early diagnosis and early treatment are essential for CLD

The early diagnosis rate of CLD is still low, which is partially due to asymptomatic phenomena and negligence of the patients. Ultrasound screening is still the first choice applicable for primary healthcare hospitals, whereas CT/MRI is more accurate but costly.

Standard follow up, as well as health awareness are vital for CLD

Regular checkups involving clinic visits and laboratory tests are able to monitor development of disease and regulate the timely use of therapies. Patients should go through complete blood counts, liver biochemistry tests, electrolyte tests, coagulation measurements, AF measurements and tests for viral loads of hepatic B virus and hepatic C viru every three months.

1.7   DESIGN GOALS FOR CLASSIFICATION OF CLD

Because of inaccuracy, insensitivity, and inspecificity challengir and interesting issues may arise on classifying the chronic liver diseas However, when integrating dynamic classifiers with the large number features set, lot of issues will arise on considering Detection Rate (DR Overall Accuracy (OA), and Processing Time (PT).

1.8   RESEARCH OBJECTIVE

This research's main objective is to design a detection mechanis for detecting and identifying the chronic liver disease from the abnorm patient and to enhance preventing them from all other diseases in an effectiv way. Essentially, the developed classifier and feature selection method shoul have the ability to find out disease in the natural way, accurate performanc prediction, accurate detection, sensitivity, specificity, and so o Consequently, at the criterion that the features selection for classificatio consuming with more number of features set and computational resources fe implementation, the developed classifier in this research work should be eas to handle as well as for performing further execution. . The proposed metho should also support the classification of chronic liver disease for attainin better performance, better efficiency, and reliability.

This research proposes a method to analyze an exclusive patholog in hierarchical basis like chronic hepatitis, compensated cirrhosis an decompensated cirrhosis. The method will be proposed with Discrimina Boundary features based on the clinical classifiers named DBFCC. The ma motivation of this research work to detect and classify the chronic liver diseases, feature selection and extraction is performed with Hough based histogram oriented gradient features and the classifier is the Markov model classifier which is used to find the staging of various conditions. Another proposed method is used to detect and classify some of the clinical features by using the Haar wavelet decomposition method. The feature extraction stage removes the unwanted non relevant data into meaningful observations. First order statistics and co-occurrence matrix Features based on statistics of texture gives far less number of relevant, non-redundant, interpretable and distinguishable features in comparison to features extracted using wavelet transformation. The proposed research work will be carried out by calculating the mean, standard deviation and mutual correlation between the images before and after extracting the features and then finally to classify the Cirrhosis and normal sized images.

1.9   PROBLEM DEFINITION

The early diagnosis rate of CLD is still low, which is partially due to asymptomatic phenomena and negligence of the patients. Liver function tests are not determined accurately. Classification approaches of different stages to CLD are inaccurate. Some of the non-invasive measurements are performed with inaccurate results. The patients with two or more mixed diseases are not identified properly. Patients are not treated with proper treatment.

The analysis is done by the invasive method to assess a liver biopsy. The results allow some hurdles such as pain after liver biopsy. For the above circumstances noninvasive methods are used as a secondary for liver biopsy. From the literature review it seems that noninvasive methods show similar accuracy with liver biopsy (Gaiani *et al.* (1997), Schuppan transient elastography (US based technology), hepascore and asparta platelet ratio index are non-invasive liver biopsy methods. Wh compared to the single method, combined methods give a better analysi But, these methods are not a better substitute biopsy since they have son limitations with absence of infrastructure. However, CLD classification d to its inaccuracy, insensitivity, inspecificity and poor detection rate has pave the way for more processing time to affect its performance.

1.10   OUR RESEARCH APPROACH

This research involves the accurate detection and classification CLD. It evolves in designing accurate multiple detection schemes against other classifiers found in CLD. A detailed description of the proposed worl is given below:

Initially, classification performance in CLD is improved t introducing a new ELM-HHOG based feature extraction. Mitigation of CL through multiple classifiers is the main goal of ELM-HHOG. Hence, multip detection schemes are created and allowed them for detecting the presence CLD as quickly as possible. Also, classification performance is obtaine further to improve overall accuracy. Notably, these multi detection classifie are better balanced and shared for both detection and classification using tl proposed mechanism; thereby, ensuring the CLD detection. To improve tl classification performance and overall accuracy, the ELM clinical classifie are used by the proposed mechanism for the creation of dynamic mul detection classifiers. In the proposed mechanism, each classification stag highly optimizes classifiers and features set by avoiding inaccura classification and drastically increasing the computer aided diagnosis in a hospitals.

From the past decades, chronic liver disease is largely focused on most of the research works. Most of them deal with detecting and identifying chronic liver disease using detection and classification approaches. But, when a single method is used to detect and classify the chronic liver disease then, these approaches cannot behave accurately and become weak in finding the diseases. Thus, the classification performance is largely degraded. However, CLD becomes harmful to the human body when fails to predict the diseases at the earliest. Thus, a mechanism called extreme learning machine and recursive feature elimination based feature selection is then developed in the second phase to enhance the conventional scheme in detecting the CLD trying to launch a collaborative method. The conventional scheme selected features may act as inaccurate showing normal behavior same as that of the pathological behavior. In order to overcome this hurdle, extreme learning machine is performed using kernel functions. Also, recursive feature elimination technique is imposed to detect the CLD and identifying them from all other diseases. However, our new proposed scheme is initiated with the following situation: the image features are selected by recursive feature elimination and further determined with radial bias function using kernel. Notably, the new proposed scheme is initiated with the above condition because, the existing method determines the classification as inaccurate and then further unable to classify the different stages of chronic liver disease. Eventually the system gets failed. The proposed method inherits the principle of conventional method, but it incorporates extreme learning machine clinical based classifier. This will help the system to identify the chronic liver disease and find out the different stages of chronic liver disease. This method discriminates healthy from pathologic conditions. To improve the ELM performance, different types of kernels such as radial basis function (RBF) and polynomial (second and third order) are applied.

A cooperative task performed in multi-level wavelet transform coefficients, in which the image features participates mainly in t coefficients of feature points. However most of the coefficients are n significant. In order to solve this problem, opening out the most freque intensity values instead of coefficients. Hence, this technique is known histogram equalization. To detect the chronic liver disease a nov unsupervised learning machine and histogram equalization based featu extraction Mechanism has been applied for ultrasound images in the thi phase. Here, the features are extracted using histogram equalization contrast approach. The core idea of this mechanism is to find out all t affected portion in given images obtained from ultrasound features. Using th proposed mechanism, only the quality of images can be improved usir image enhancement technique. Moreover, the interest area from the bac ground of the image is segmented using k means clustering algorithr Finally Haar wavelet decomposition is used to classify the different stages CLD. The classification performance of proposed approaches is analyze using certain important factors such as, accuracy, sensitivity and specificit Through quantitative evaluation, it is observed that the extreme learnir machine and recursive feature elimination based feature selection methc attains high accuracy compared to other proposed object approaches.

1.11   RESEARCH CONTRIBUTIONS

This thesis's central objective is to portray the design ar development of efficient based detecting schemes for the classification CLD. The proposed methods focused mainly on sustainability in a dynam environment, improving performance, and attaining better accuracy. Th valuable contributions of this thesis are described below.

1.   ELM-HHOG based Feature Extraction

- To improve the performance and overall accuracy, an ensemble learning machine and Hough histogram oriented gradient based feature extraction for the classification of CLD has been developed to exploits the dynamic multi detection classifiers to handle the edge of the region in the image.

- Combined classifiers are used fully to develop many feature selection classifiers as far as possible, so that classifiers can quickly detect the CLD and its stages; hence achieved better overall accuracy and detection rate.

2.   ELM-RFE based Feature Selection

Next, the ELM-RFE method is introduced in this dissertation for the classification of CLD that include the following:

- To detect and classify the CLD with the help of multiple classifiers colluding together in the classification performance called collaborative method, a new ELM-RFE based feature selection Scheme is introduced. The features are selected by recursive feature elimination method.

- Second order, Third order and Polynomial using kernel function with radial bias function are developed in ELM-RFE to detect and classify CLD from other diseases. In other words, this method inherits the principle of the conventional method, but it incorporates extreme learning machine clinical based classifier. This will help the system identify the chronic liver disease and determine the different stages of chronic liver disease.

3.   **ULM-HE based Feature Extraction**

- To classify the CLD a novel unsupervised learning machine and histogram equalization based feature extraction has been applied. A new model ULM clinical based classifier is used to detect and classify the disease in an effective manner.

- The core idea of this mechanism is to find out the entire affected portion in given image obtained from ultrasound features. Using this proposed mechanism, Morphological Haar wavelet decomposition is used to classify the different stages of CLD.

1.12   OUTLINE OF THE THESIS

Chapter 1 deliberates a brief introduction to the entire research outline and explains the novelties relayed in the research.

Chapter 2 describes a brief review of existing research contributions. Each and every research contribution's essence created by the scholars in the previous years is presented.

Chapter3 describes the proposed **Ensemble Learning Machine** and **Hough Histogram Oriented Gradient** based **Feature Extraction for Classification of CLD**. It uses an efficient detection mechanism that exploits the dynamic multi detection classifiers to handle the edge of the region in the image and improve classification performance.

Chapter 4 explains the proposed **Extreme Learning Machine** and **Recursive Feature Elimination** based **Feature selection for Classification of CLD**. The proposed module handles different models to improve the classification performance.

Chapter 5 explains the proposed **Unsupervised Learning Machine** and **Histogram Equalization** based **Feature Extraction for Classification of CLD.** The proposed module handles different schemes to improve classification performance. Also, the comparative analysis of the three proposed methods is provided in this chapter.

Chapter 6 provides an overall research conclusion and scope of future research.

CHAPTER 2

ANALYSIS OF CHRONIC LIVER DISEASE

Intelligent procedures based on backgrounds have played a vibrant role in liver disease finding. From statistical techniques to image processing algorithms and image processing algorithms to deep learning methods, all these methods have been commonly deployed on liver investigation data for estimating the sickness. Due to increasing vagueness and complexities in the datasets, deriving comprehensible information becomes the main challenge for clinicians. Here are some of the methods which are used to detect and classify the image based on feature selection.

2.1   INTRODUCTION

Minhas *et al.* (2012) proposed the work based on the ROI method to partially extract the region of interest. In this method some of the region of interest were extracted manually and they were trained in the identification of liver disease with fewer human interventions.

Andrade *et al.* (2012) proposed a semi-automatic method of classification to recognize fatty liver by implementing the textural feature with higher order statistical analysis. This researcher has calculated the accuracy with k mean classifier and improved the classification accuracy to 78%.

Virmani *et al.* (2013) proposed an automated system for normal cirrhotic carcinoma using the text descriptors. The accuracy of the classification was made with the help of WPT text descriptors to extract the mean and standard deviation and energy features. By implementing this method, the accuracy has been increased to **88.8 %**.

Wu et al. (2013) proposed a system based on the fusion system's hierarchical features for ultrasonic liver tissue. The features were selected for the classification of ultrasonic liver tissue. In this method, a KNN classifier was used; by implementing this method, the accuracy of 95.05% was achieved.

Yang *et al.* (2014) proposed a classification method to classify pathological images based on voting. The unique model was developed to optimize statistical analysis to obtain better performance.

Owjimehar *et al.* (2015) proposed an improved method for liver diseases .The method was able to select the regions of interest in the liver images. A two-level wavelet packet transforms analyzed these optimum regions of interest. The features were extracted from some statistical features. Support vector machine and k-nearest neighbor classifiers were used to classify the images. Compared to all other classifier the Support vector machine attained the accuracy of 97.9%.

Owimeh *et al.* (2017) proposed a Staging of Fatty Liver Diseases Based on Hierarchical Classification and Feature Fusion. In this method back-scan conversion of ultrasound sector images was used. This method was based on a hierarchical classification. The approach was performed into two processes. The first process selected the optimum regions of interest from the focal zone of the given ultrasound images. In the second process, normal and fatty liver was performed on hierarchical basis. The features were extracted using the wavelet packet transform and gray-level co-occurrence matrix. A support vector machine classifier was used to distinguish between normal and fatty liver. The results of this method clearly illustrated the efficiency of the system with an overall accuracy of 94.91%

Ilias *et al.* (2017) proposed a Machine-Learning Algorithm for Chronic Liver Disease using Ultrasound Shear Wave Elastography. The purpose of this method was to design a computer-aided diagnosis system which classifies chronic liver disease. The clustering and machine-learning algorithms were used. Stepwise regression was used for feature reduction. support vector machine was used to classify the chronic liver disease from healthy cases and 87.3 % accuracy was achieved.

Puja *et al.* (2018) proposed a classification of chronic liver disease based on ultrasound images. The features were extracted by using a grey-level difference matrix. Moreover, feature fusion schemes were implemented. The combination of the Relief filter method and the sequential forward selection wrapper method was used to classify the liver stages. A computer-aided system was designed to classify liver conditions. In this method forward central and backward was used. The performance of this method was compared with previous feature extraction methods. The experiment studies were carried out by 754 ultrasound images. The accuracy of 94.5% was obtained.

Karan agarwal *et al.* (2019) proposed a method for detection of cirrhosis in ultrasound images using intensity difference technique. The method was used to distinguish the cirrhotic liver from normal liver. The features were extracted by using the region of interest. The intensity difference technique was used. This method's analysis was done on 8 cirrhotic images and 30 normal liver images, and the classification accuracy of 98.18% was achieved.

Many researchers have developed many detection and classification tools against chronic liver disease. In this module, different feature extraction methods and various classifiers are studied and analyzed.

2.2   SURVEY ON ULTRASOUND IMAGING

Ultrasound imaging is a broadly used technology for the diagnosis of liver diseases. Ultrasound imaging is a popular and noninvasive method frequently used in the diagnoses of liver diseases. The computer-aided system is used to classify the normal, fatty, and heterogeneous liver by analyzing the textural features of Ultrasound images.

Table 2.1 Literal works on Ultrasound Imaging

S. No	Reference	Textural Features	Classifier	Disease	Accuracy %
1	Kyriacou *et al.* (1997)	GLDS, RUNL, SGLDM, FDTA	KNN	Normal, Fatty, Cirrhosis	82.2
2	Lee *et al.*(2003)	FFVBWT	H	Normal, Cirrhosis, Hepatoma	96.7
3	Yeh *et al.*(2005)	GLCM, NSWT	SVM	Steatosis, Non Steatosis	90.5
4	Ribeiro *et al.*(2009)	SIF,DIF	B	Normal,Fatty	95
5	Sirui *et al.*(2010)	WPT	SVM	Normal, Cirrhosis	85.79
6	Ricardo *et al.*(2011)	SIF,DIF	SVM,DT, KNN	Chronic liver disease	73.20

Table 2.1 (Continued)

S. No	Reference	Textural Features	Classifier	Disease	Accura %‌
7	Wu et al.(2012)	OA,GA	A	Liver Cirrhosis	Not Give
8	Acharya et al.(2012)	HOS,DWT	DT	Liver disease	93.3
9	Ricardo et al.(2012)	CBC	H	Hepatic disease	Not Give
10	Andreia et al.(2012)	SR	ANN,SVM, KNN	Steototic liver disease	High
11	Wu et al.(2013)	HFF	KNN	Liver tissue	95.05
12	Suganya et al.(2013)	GLCM	SVM	Fatty, Cirrhosis	Not Give
13	Hemia et al.(2014)	GLCM	LIBSVM	Liver disease	96.5
14	Owjimehar et al. (2015)	WPT	SVM,KNN	Normal, Fatty, Heterogeneous	97.9
15	Owimeh et al.(2016)	GLCM, OROI, BSCWPT	SVM	Normal, Fatty	94.91
16	Usman et al.(2016)	CAC,CM,CH	SVM	Normal, Abnormal	83
17	Ilias et al.(2017)	CA,MLA	SVM	Chronic liver disease	87.3
18	Aman et al.(2017)	MLA	KNN	Liver disease	Not Give
19	Puja et al.(2018)	GLDM	RFSFSWM	Chronic liver,	94.5

Table 2.1 (Continued)

S. No	Reference	Textural Features	Classifier	Disease	Accuracy %
				Cirrhosis, Hepatocellular Carcinoma	
20	Nazmum *et al.* (2018)	DM	DT	Liver disease	70.67
21	Sendren *et al.*(2018)	GLCM, GLRLM, SBS,SFS	SVM	Hepatocellular Carcinoma	88.75
22	Karan *et al.*(2019)	ROI,IDT	SVM	Cirrhotic, Normal	98.18
23	Qiang *et al.*(2019)	ML,DL	CNN	Liver disease	Not Given
24	Sendren *et al.*(2019)	GLCM, GLRLM, SBS,SFS	SVM	Hepatocellular Carcinoma	88.87
25	Anand *et al.*(2019)	CBC	MPSO	Liver disease	95.4

2.2.1   Discussions on Ultrasound Imaging

Ultrasound features were used to detect the normal, fatty, and cirrhosis (Kyriacou *et al.* (1997)). The features were extracted using four different processes. The process used namely gray level difference statistics, gray level run length statistics, spatial gray level dependence matrices and fractal dimension texture analysis. The KNN classifier was used to classify the disease and obtained 82.2% accuracy. The US liver images were used to detect the liver that was normal, cirrhosis, and hepatoma (Lee *et al.* (2003)).

The features were extracted by fractal feature vector based on wavelet transform. Hierarchical classifier was used and obtained 96.7% accuracy.

Ultrasound image was used to distinguish steatosis and non steatosis liver (Yeh *et al.* (2005)). The features were extracted by gray level co-occurrence matrix (GLCM) and non-separable wavelet transform. Support vector machine (SVM) was used to classify the features, and an accuracy of 90.5% was obtained. The images were extracted from the signal generated by the US probe (Ribeiro *et al.* (2009)). The images were speckle image and despeckled image. The despeckle images filter was used to find the intensity features, and speckle images filter was used to find the texture features. Bayes classifier was used to classify the liver and 95% accuracy was obtained.US liver images were used to differentiate the cirrhosis and normal (Sirui *et al.* (2010)). By using WPT, features were extracted. The SVM classifier was used to classify the liver disease and obtained 85.79% accuracy.

Ultrasound features were used with clinical and laboratorial data to determine staging process (Ricardo *et al.* (2011)). The images were speckle image and despeckle image. The three classifiers namely SVM, KNN, DT were performed and obtained accuracy of 73.20%. US features were extracted by merging of higher-order statistics and discrete wavelet transform (Acharya *et al.* (2012)). The Accuracy of 93.3% was achieved by decision tree classifier for the normal and abnormal liver. The features were selected from the gray level co-occurrence matrix (GLCM) with 12 haralick features to classify the liver into fatty and cirrhosis (Suganya *et al.* (2013)). The images were preprocessed by using the Anisotropic Diffusion speckle reduction method. The obtained results from features depend on parameter namely contrast, auto correlation, Angular Second Momentum, cluster shade and cluster prominence. Support Vector Machine classifiers show that the classification accuracy rate is comparatively better than other methods

LIBSVM was used for classification to classify the liver diseases (Hamia *et al.* (2014)). This method focused on five different types of diseases. They are namely carcinoma, cirrhosis, fatty livers, hepatitis and cystic liver. Accurate classifications were done by using preprocessing and feature extraction. Feature extraction was done using a gray level and co-occurrence matrix (GLCM). This method performed liver identification in terms of accuracy and execution time.

Ultrasonic imaging is increasingly becoming useful in detecting problems and processing methods in digital image processing (Usman *et al.* (2016)). Liver diseases are caused by the liver's improper functioning that leads to various liver diseases if not predicted earlier. The automated system was implemented for normal and abnormal liver samples detection. Features selection was based on texture and color properties of ultrasonic images. In classification, SVM classifier with Radial basis function was used to classify the abnormal liver images. The Performance was analyzed and 83% accuracy achieved. Liver diseases are a major health problem among worldwide. Machine learning ML algorithms were used to diagnose liver disease (Aman singh *et al.* (2017)). KNN and PCA-KNN were combined together for classification. The algorithm did not show best results for all types of datasets and combined methods were not performed better than the individuals. None of the algorithm was perfect and performance of an algorithm depends on the dataset type and structure, number of observations, dimensions and decision boundary. The classification between Liver diseases and Hepatocellular Carcinoma is the most common type of liver cancer based on ultrasound image texture features and Support Vector Machine classifier (Sendren *et al.* (2018)). The features were extracted using the Gray-Level Co-occurrence Matrix and Gray-Level Run Length Matrix from the region of interests (ROIs) in ultrasound images. The Three feature selection models namely Sequential Forward Selection, Sequential Backward

Selection, F-score, were used to determine the identification of the liv
diseases. The classification of HCC and liver abscess was done by SVM wi
the accuracy of 88.75%.

2.2.2   Inference based on the Survey of Ultrasound Imaging

For accurate identification and classification of Chronic liv
disease, medical experts prefer Ultrasound images that satisfy its bas
requirements such as accuracy, detection rate, overall accuracy, mea
standard deviation and mutual correlation while performing the operation
On the other hand, these methods are preferred because of the performance
detecting liver diseases (i.e. due to the severe problem such as pain, bleedir
and so on. for such situations, finding the diseases at the earlier stage wi
reduce the death rate). However, in this chapter, a survey is conducted c
Ultrasound imaging proposed by various researchers to analyze th
effectiveness and performance while performing the detection ar
classification of CLD. The performance has been analysed using differe
parameters such as accuracy, sensitivity and reliability.

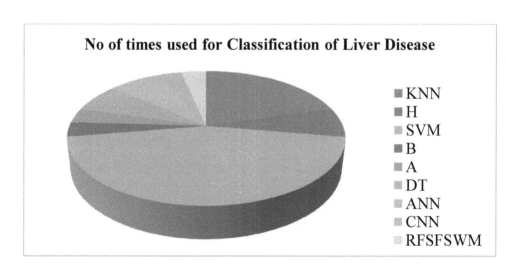

Figure 2.1 Classifier used for Ultrasound based Image

From the above survey, it can be observed that the Ultrasound imaging based method achieved maximum accuracy because most of the conventional method based Ultrasound imaging for identification and classification is done by efficient feature selection method. From the survey (Figure 2.1), the Ultrasound imaging based method on medical diagnosis for identifying and staging of the liver disease using classifiers achieves higher accuracy by Support Vector Machine (13 times), K-Nearest neighbor (6 times) and so on. By the fact, the more potentially Ultrasound imaging based method should attain 90% accuracy. The above studied traditional ultrasound imaging based method (in Table 2.1) attained maximum detection rate, maximum accuracy and minimum classifier because; high computational strategy is experienced with the use of Ultrasound imaging that involves textural features, classifiers and additional computations. Also, Ultrasound imaging is increased in so many hospitals for the detection of diseases. Ultrasound imaging based detection method works only after getting useful information about the disease and then only proceeds for detecting chronic liver diseases. These issues mentioned in the above literature review are effectively resolved using several computational intelligence techniques that can adjust the run time and reduce the risk factor of diseases in the environments.

2.3   SURVEY ON COMPUTED TOMOGRAPHY IMAGING

In order to determine the nature of diseases (i.e. suspected or normal), the computational intelligence techniques like filters, fuzzy logic and neural network schemes are used by the computed tomography imaging based method. However, for a particular period of time, useful information regarding the disease is carried out. Computed tomography is another method for diagnosing the liver disease. In worldwide, cancer is the fifth reason for death factor; therefore, detection and classification of liver diseases have great significance because of its widespread. There are several types of diseases which liver cancer is the third position for death factor. This cancer is also called as hepatic disease. This type of disease starts from the liver and the grows further if not diagnosed early. The disease which starts from oth organ in the human body and travels to liver is not treated as liver diseases. liver disease consists of the hepatic growths called tumors over liver or insic liver. Therefore, early detection of liver disease is a challenging task i practical radiology. There are so many numbers of computer aided diagnost methods designed using image processing methods for early accura detection. Early stage detection of liver disease helps to prevent it completel through the proper treatment. The major issues with image processing base methods are efficiency, processing time and accuracy of detection. Designin time efficient, high accuracy and simple detection method is the leadin research problem. The threshold values are justified by checking if th threshold falls within the same value estimated for each image. Th contributes by providing a computer aided diagnostic system for the diagnos of the liver disease using CT images. Results are evaluated with medic radiologists.

Table 2.2 Literal works on Computed Tomography Imaging

S.No	Reference	Textural Features	Classifier	Disease	Accuracy %
1	Gletsos et al. (2001)	IDM, SFFS	FFNN	Normal,Hepatic, Hemangioma, HCC	98
2	Gletsos et al. (2003)	GLCM, SFFS,GA	FFNN	Normal,Hepatic, Hemangioma, HCC	97

Table 2.2 (Continued)

S.No	Reference	Textural Features	Classifier	Disease	Accuracy %
3	Mougiakakou *et al.* (2003)	FOS, SGLDM, GLDM,GA	4NNBPA	Normal,Hepatic, Hemangioma, HCC	97
4	Mala *et al.* (2006)	BWT	LVQ	Benign, HCC	92
5	Mougiakakou *et al.* (2007)	FOS, SGLDM, GLDM,GA	5MPNN	Normal,Hepatic, Hemangioma, HCC	84.96
6	Wang *et al.* (2009)	FOS,SGLDM, GLDM, GLRLM	MSVM	Normal, Hemangioma, HCC	97.78
7	Mala *et al.* (2010)	BWSTF, SFFS,GA	PNN,LVQ, BPN	Fatty liver, Cirrhosis	PNN-96 LVQ-93 BPN-80
8	Kumar *et al.* (2010)	FDCT	FFNN	Hemangioma, HCC	93.3
9	Gunasundari *et al.* (2012)	CM,FDCT	BPN,PNN, CFBPN	Hemangioma, HCC	96
10	Kumar *et al.* (2012)	GLFOS, GLCM, CCFOS, CCCMPCA	PNN	Hemangioma, HCC	GLFOS-79 GLCM-86 CCFOS-93 CCCM-94
11	Priyanka *et al.*(2014)	FL	NN	Liver diseases	Not Given
12	Alyaa *et al.* (2015)	HFOS	KM	Liver diseases	Not Given

Table 2.2 (Continued)

S.No	Reference	Textural Features	Classifier	Disease	Accuracy %
13	Vitoantonio et al.(2017)	ROI, MA	NN	HCC	Not Given
14	Ignisha et al. (2019)	WOASA	SVM, KNN,RF	Chronic Liver disease	98

2.3.1 Discussions on Computed Tomography Imaging

Sequential forward floating selection and inverse differenc moment were the two different methods used to detect and identify of th liver disease using CT images (Gletsos et al. (2001)). The feed forward neur. network classifier was used to classify the liver disease. The performance wa analyzed by obtaining an accuracy of 98%. The features were selecte continuously using different metho namely sequential forward floating and genetic algorithm. Based on th behavior, diseases were classified using a feed forward neural netwo (Gletsos et al. (2003)). Further, an analysis was performed based on the da collected from the scan center.

Liver diseases that behaved in a suspected manner were detecte using first order statistics with a 4 class propagation model. The gray lev dependent matrix and spatial Gray level depende matrix was used to detect the diseases using the feature extraction techniq (Mougiakakou et al. (2003)). To analyze the performance, the diseases we classified by means of a neural network classifier. Chronic liver diseases we monitored continuously by CT images (Mala et al. (2006)).In case, if foun any variations in the behavior of diseases then that diseases were marked malignant. After marking the diseases for a number of times (i.e. attains certain accuracy) then that disease is considered as a Hepatocellular Carcinoma.

Using CT images, the diseases were monitored in the features set by applying first order statistics with a Multilayer perceptron neural network model. The gray level dependent matrix and spatial Gray level dependent matrix were used to detect the diseases using the feature extraction technique (Mougiakakou *et al.* (2007)). To analyze the performance, the diseases were identified using a multilayer classifier. The gray level run length matrix was applied to find out the liver diseases. As similar to the above said method, the diseases were continuously monitored using the multi support vector machine classifier (Wang *et al.* (2009)).

By taking into account of the performance, the diseases were classified in a probabilistic neural network classifier. Detection and classification were done simultaneously using the sequential forward floating method (Mala *et al.* (2010)). Conversely, diseases were classified by Bayes classifier. A special monitoring method was involved in fast discrete curvelet transform to monitor the other diseases forwarding activities (Kumar *et al.* (2010)).

The co-occurrence matrix and fast discrete curvelet transform mechanism were used for detect the liver diseases and give the proper treatment for the diseases in the earlier stage (Gunasundari *et al.* (2012)). The cascade feed forward BPN was used for the classification of liver diseases. Diseases were isolated from the scan centre using CT images. Conversely, disease was classified by using promiscuous probabilistic neural network classifier. A monitoring method was involved in contour let first order statistics algorithm to monitor the disease stage (Kumar *et al.* (2012)).

Another algorithm for liver disease detection was based on fuzzy logic and neural network (Priyanka et al. (2014)). Neuro-fuzzy systems were suitable tools for extracting useful information from images. In this method, the liver disease was detected through the CT images in three phases: the pre-processing phase, the processing phase, and the detection phase. Initially, the pre-processing phase, a set of medical images was filtered for removing unwanted noise. Then the filtered image was segmented using fuzzy logic and neural network. In the detection, part neurofuzzified segmented CT images were registered to obtain the disease. The result was obtained for a few different sets of data set. The segmentation process was based on the hybrid method, which combines the modified k-Mean classifier and the first-order statistical. The computed tomography features were used to extract the region's boundary in the liver image and further classify the stages of liver diseases (Alyaa et al. (2015)).

Computer-Aided Decision (CAD) systems based on Medical Imaging support radiologists in finding the Hepatocellular carcinoma (HCC) using Computed Tomography (CT) images by avoiding invasive medical procedures such as biopsies (Vitoantonio et al. (2017)). Several approaches were implemented to segment the region of the liver using the ROI method. At the end of the preprocessing phases, the features were extracted by means of morphological process and proposed an evolutionary algorithm to optimize neural network classifiers based on different subsets of features. noninvasive approach for detecting chronic liver disease was proposed using the classifiers' ensemble learning machine (Ignisha et al. (2019)). The whale minimization algorithm with simulated annealing was used for feature selection which is used to classify chronic liver disease accurately. Ensemble classifiers consist of a support vector machine, k—Nearest Neighbor, and the random forest were used to classify the stages of liver diseases. The feature selected using the whale optimization algorithm with simulated annealing improved the classification performance. The liver classification using ensemble classifier achieved 98% accuracy.

2.3.2 Inference based on the Survey of Computed Tomography Imaging

Instead of using the medical images by ultrasound imaging, medical images are used by the computed tomography imaging. Many times if a disease is marked as malignant then that disease is considered as a liver disease.

From the aforementioned study, several advantages of using neural network classifier on CLD were observed and they are described as follows:

a) The terms of accuracy indicate the performance of neural network classifier. Moreover, neural network is incorporated using the knowledge derived from the network field.

b) To design a neural network classifier it is not so much essential to make a mathematical analysis of the system. However, it is hard to create a mathematical analysis for the system and if it is not applicable to the CLD then, data set of features is considered by this system.

c) The neural network classifier classifies the disease by analyzing the performance in terms of accuracy. The neural network classifier system is handled efficiently, easily and finally correct classification is made.

d) Essentially, compared to the other computational intelligence methods the neural network classifier exhibits less execution time, maximum efficiency, maximum detection rate, sensitivity, reliability and more flexibility.

The aforementioned goodness of neural network classifier showed that classification could be done effectively without any difficulty.

However, the efficiency of computed tomography imaging for CLD and applying neural network on CT imaging for the detection and classification is analyzed. From the survey (Figure 2.2), it is observed that when applying neural network classifier for the detection and classification of liver disease, it showed more satisfactory performance (in terms of accuracy, efficiency, and sensitivity) than the other classifier scheme .This is because the neural network classifier on CT imaging can adjust the time and critical situations. Also, these techniques when embedded on multi layer classifier can largely support the detection and classification of CLD.

Moreover, from the aforementioned study (in Table 2.2) it observed that the traditional extraction methods adopting computed tomography image for the detection has increased the computational level and classification is done by applying all the classifiers in all the data set of features due to the information given by CT images. Moreover, the CT image allows rapid processing. CT image examinations are feasible with reduced computation time. CT image can efficiently be used to detect liver disease irrespective of their size, shape, density, and heterogeneity within short running time (half a minute). The performances indicate that the tool provide the level of freedom that is enough to solve real clinical problems.

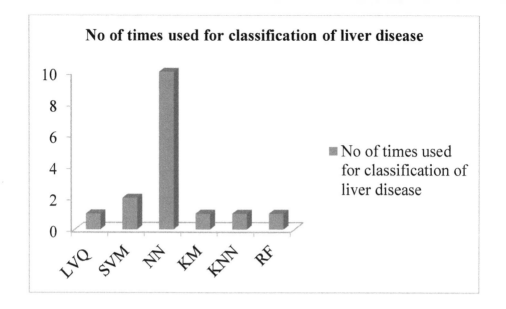

Figure 2.2 Classifier used for Computed Tomography based Image

However, these problems mentioned in the above literature review for detection and classification can be resolved effectively through employing a multi-layer classifiers scheme in the prior works rather than applying network classifier for the detection of disease. Thus, the overall efficiency of the classifier is increased and overall specificity will also be increased in the approaches as mentioned above. Moreover, the survey carried out to determine the goodness of using MRI imaging rather than adopting CT imaging is shown below.

2.4 SURVEY ON MAGNETIC RESONANCE IMAGING

MR Imaging is one of the imaging tests for liver disease detection and classification and this modality provides high resolution to liver contrast. MR imaging does not use ionizing radiation. The main advantages of MR Imaging include a high resolution, better sensitivity, better detection and classification than with CT, and lack of ionizing radiation. MR Imaging can safely be used with patients by iodinated contrast agents. The main drawbacks of MR Imaging include high cost, a long time and the need for the patient to hold their breath for longer. Contrast techniques are usually employed in M imaging. This technique is adopted to monitor all the affecting area in th liver. This scheme mostly achieves better performance due to the deploymer of the contrast technique for the entire MR image remaining in the data se Due to this fact, the cost is more on finding the disease in the MR imag Features set in the MR image to share the information for the determination c CLD. A false statement can be easily avoided using the MR image. In oth words, maximum performance is achieved by the efficient technique M image.

Table 2.3 Literal works on Magnetic Resonance Imaging

S.No	Reference	Textural Features	Classifier	Disease	Accurac %
1	Jayant et al. (2008)	Diffusion weight imaging	MR Elastography	Hepatic, Fibrosis	Not Giver
2	Bachir et al. (2009)	Diffusion, Perfusion weight imaging	MR Spectrography	Hepatic, HCC	Not Giver
3	Yehonatan et al. (2011)	Machine Learning, Statistical Model	MSVM	Liver Fibrosis	78
4	Zhiming et al. (2015)	Diffusion, Perfusion weight imaging	ECM	Liver Fibrosis	Not Given
5	Leonie et al. (2016)	Image based Technique, Morphologic	Elastography	Liver Fibrosis	Not Given

Table 2.3 (Continued)

S.No	Reference	Textural Features	Classifier	Disease	Accuracy %
6	Zhenjiang *et al.*(2017)	GLCM, GLGCM, GLRLM, GWTF	KNN, BP-ANN, SVM	Hepatic, Haemangioma, HCC	Not Given
7	Petitclerc *et al.*(2017)	Diffusion weight imaging	MR Elastography	Liver Fibrosis, HCC	Not Given
8	Hykoush *et al.* (2019)	Morphologic Features Extraction	Contours	Pancreas	Not Given
9	Asuka *et al.* (2019)	Machine Learning Model	Topological Data analysis	Hepatic, Haemangioma, HCC	92

2.4.1 Discussions on Magnetic Resonance Imaging

A Method which includes magnetic resonance spectroscopy, diffusion-weighted MR, and MR Elastography was used for detecting the fibrosis (Jayant *et al.* (2008)). Compared to other non-invasive methods, MR imaging provides the functional and biological information about hepatic fibrosis and further gives proper treatment for hepatic fibrosis. Diffusion and Perfusion weight imaging was co-operated together for detection of hepatic disease (Bachiret *et al.* (2009)). Then, this co-operated information was used to classify the disease using MR Spectrography.

A machine-learning approach was used for the interactive classification of liver disease, and also for the automatic classification and staging of liver fibrosis (Yehonatan *et al.* (2011)).The classification of suspected metastasis uses statistical modelling to classify the hepatic disease and follow their early hemodynamical changes. Changes in hepatic were evaluated from MR images. A classification model was done to distinguish between the healthy and pathologic conditions. The classification of the liver fibrosis was performed with a hierarchical multiclass binary based support vector machine (SVM) classifier. Most probably, in clinical practice, patient may reject additional liver biopsies because of the long-term follow-up (Zhiming *et al.* (2015)). To resolve these problems, a number of different noninvasive methods have been developed for the accurate diagnosis of liver fibrosis. A new approach was developed for accurately diagnosing early-stage liver fibrosis. During that stage the disease may be cured by active treatment. The image-based technique (Leonie et al. (2016)) extracts features in which the morphological approach made a feature selection, and the classification of liver fibrosis was done using Elastography based on MR images.

In another method, the Feature analysis was performed from the different schemes like gray level co-occurrence matrix, gray level gradient co-occurrence matrix, gray level run length matrix, Gabor wavelet transform, intensity size zone matrix and histogram features (Zhenjiang *et al.* (2017)). Four classifiers were trained with the features set in the classification of disease types.MRI based techniques for liver fibrosis were used to find the disease of liver fibrosis. The MRI-based technique includes magnetic resonance elastography, diffusion-weighted imaging, texture analysis, perfusion imaging, hepatocellular function assessment, strain imaging and $T_{1\rho}$ imaging (Petitclerc *et al.* (2017)). For each technique, provided a general discussion of the physical concept, and analyze their diagnostic performance

A method was used to determine the accuracy for classification of hepatic disease which includes the classification of T1-weighted Magnetic Resonance (MR) images using machine learning models approaches (Asuka *et al.* (2019)). Texture analysis and topological data analysis were performed using persistent homology. For classification, texture features were calculated. Our methods using texture analysis or topological data analysis allowed for classification of the hepatic disease with considerable accuracy, was useful when applied for computer-aided diagnosis with MR images. A novel approach for automatic pancreas segmentation is magnetic resonance imaging (MRI) scans (Hykoush *et al.* (2019)). This method was used for 3D segmentation and also combined with geometrical and morphological analysis for the classification of the abdominal tissue. Distinct contours in tight pixel range did the classification.

2.4.2   Inference based on the Survey of Magnetic Resonance Imaging

From the aforementioned study (in Table 2.3.), it is observed that the MR imaging-based detection method could accurately diagnose the disease. Notably, the combined schemes show texture features and texture parameters have computational complexity with the additional features set for making calculations.

Moreover, after evaluating with the parameters such as accuracy, sensitivity and specificity, the MR imaging based scheme exhibited a satisfactory performance on finding the types of diseases through the combining above mentioned technique. This goodness is because the MR imaging based approach due to its classification performance captures all the attention of other classifier schemes.

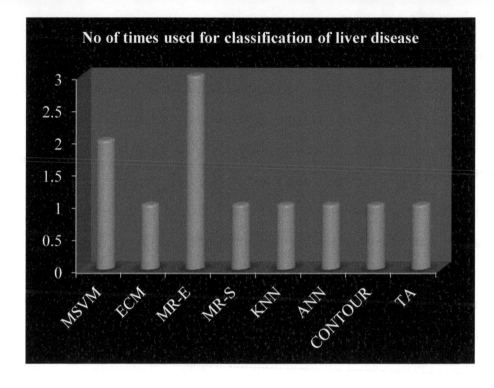

Figure 2.3 Classifier used for Magnetic Resonance based Image

From the aforementioned study (in Table 2.3), it is observed th
the traditional MR imaging- based scheme that is used for detecting the liv
disease have attained satisfactory accuracy and overall performance is bett
compared to the above discussed schemes. Also, when evaluated wit
parameters such as, accuracy, sensitivity and specificity the MR imagir
based scheme shows satisfactory performance and the classifier used fo
classification of liver disease as shown in (figure 2.3). However, thes
problems mentioned in the above literature review for the detection an
classification can be resolved effectively through employing multi layo
classifiers scheme in the prior works rather than applying single classifier fo
the detection of disease. Thus, the overall efficiency of classifier becomo
better and overall specificity will also be better in the above mentiono
approaches. Moreover, the survey carried out to determine the goodness o
using MRI imaging.

2.5   SURVEY ON VARIOUS FEATURE EXTRACTION METHODS

The features used to determine a subset of the inceptive features is called feature selection. The selected features are anticipated to contain the relevant information from the input data, so that the task can be performed by using make less delineation instead of the complete data. Feature extraction is a process of converting the given data into a set of occurrence points.

2.5.1   Discussions on Various Feature Extraction Methods

Table 2.4 Literal works on Feature Extraction based scheme

Sl. no	Reference	Proposed method	Application	Limitation
1.	Raksha *et al.* (2017)	Histogram of Oriented Gradients	Detecting the objects	More time to extract
2	Herbert Bay *et al.* (2017)	Speeded-Up Robust Features	Object recognition	High dimensionality
3	Karan Agarwal *et al.* (2016)	Local Binary Patterns	Statistical and structural models of texture analysis	Slow down the recognition speed especially on big data set
4	Ricardo *et al.* (2013)	Haar Wavelets	Decomposition and reconstruction	Not continuous
5	Mendonça *et al.* (2017)	Color Histograms	Image Processing	Ignoring shape and texture

The histogram of oriented gradients is a feature descriptor used in image processing to detect the objects. This method counts the occurrence of gradient orientation in localized portions of an image. Raksha *et al.* (201? proposed an approach based on the HOG feature, to get the HOG feature. The edges portion was extracted from the images. The edge detection tool was used to achieve this objective. Spatial layout information plays a vital role. Each image was divided into a sequence of spatial grids by doubling the number of divisions in each axis direction so that each dimension has cell. Before the HOG feature was formed, there was another variable that needs to be done (i.e.) for counting the histogram of edge orientations. The number of orientations was sampled into K-bins. Each bin in the histogram delineated the number of edges with orientations over certain angular period.

Speeded up robust features is a local feature detector and descriptor. It can be used for jobs such as object recognition, image registration, classification and 3D reconstruction. The Scale Invariant Feature Transform descriptor partly links it. Herbert Bay *et al.* (2017) developed novel approach for Speeded up Robust Features. This method performed with a scale and rotation invariant for the detector and descriptor. This method outperformed much faster than existing methods with respect to repeatability, distinctiveness and robustness. This work was achieved by integrating the images using image convolutions and thus leading to a combination of detection, description and matching steps.

It is used to marks the pixels of an image by thresholding the area of each pixel. It generates the output as a binary number. Due to its performance, Local Binary Pattern texture operator has become a popular method in various applications. It can be used for the statistical and structural grayscale image to mean weighted grayscale. Reproduction of the ultrasound image on the fundamental of local binary patterns method was applied to various texture patterns detection. Local Binary Pattern was initially proposed for texture analysis(Karan Agarwal*et al.* (2016)). This method was used to detect and classify the liver cirrhosis based on texture pattern from the US images. During the past years, Local Binary Pattern raised increasing in the field of medical image processing. Otsu method is a process of changing grayscale image to a binary image using adaptive thresholding. OTSU was additionally added with Local Binary Pattern which generates weighted gray scale image and so Local Binary Pattern is called modified Local Binary Pattern. The modified Local Binary Pattern method is termed as a differential local binary pattern.

Haar wavelet is a process of rescaling like square shape basis which together forms a wavelet function .Wavelet analysis is similar to the Fourier analysis which allows a targeted basis over an interval period. This can be represented in terms of an orthonormal basis. The wavelets transform method was used for decomposing and reconstructing images using the digital filter technique (Ricardo *et al.* (2013)). Digital filter contains low pass and high pass filters. The low pass filter output includes the overall shape of the signal, and so it is called approximation. The high pass filter output includes vertical, horizontal and diagonal components. Moreover, the wavelet transform divides the image into four bands (images) called wavelet decomposition process. In order to reconstruct the image, the inverse wavelet transform is used. The original signal is reconstructed using inverse LPF and inverse HPF.

In image processing, a color histogram is a delineation of the distribution of colors in an image. For the digital images, a color histogram

Color Histogram is the technique used for the feature extraction in the retrieval of color based image. Color Histogram is a method for showing the color content of the image (i.e.) counting the number of pixel of each color. The work done by Mendonça *et al.* (2017) stated the use of color histogram for evaluating the joint destruction, and then applying histogram as a technique to classify the affected region into different three grades like Grade 0, Grade 1, Grade 2 and Grade 3 based on the seriousness of the disease.

2.5.2 Inference based on the Survey of Feature Extraction Methods

Moreover, the various feature extraction methods are already discussed in the above literature review (in Table 2.4). The methods are

- Gray Level Difference Statistics

- Spatial Gray Level Dependence Matrices

- Gray Level Run Length Matrix

- Gray Level Histogram

- Texture Energy Measure

- First Order Statistics

- Gray Level Co-occurrence Matrices

Statistics are the gray level of first-order statistics and second order statistics. The gray level difference elaborates the spatial relationship between image pixels. First-order statistics are determined from original image values. In second-order statistics, the image properties fall on pixel pairs. Spatial gray level dependence matrices are the statistical method for finding a texture that follows the spatial relationship of pixels. Spatial information is the gray-level co-occurrence matrix and also known as the gray level spatial dependence matrix.

Gray level run length matrix provides the size of equivalent runs for each grey level. This matrix is computed for the 13 different directions in the 3D image. For each 11 texture indices obtained from this matrix, the 3D value is the average for the above 13 directions. The grey level shows the brightness of a pixel. The least grey level is 0. A grey level histogram points out that how many pixels of an image share the same grey level. The x-axis indicates the grey levels (i.e. from 0 to 255), and the y-axis specify the frequency.

One of the most famous methods for texture feature analysis is the Texture Energy Measure. This method is used for detecting the edges, levels, waves, spots and ripples by taking predefined covers to the images. The first order statistic is the least sample value, once the values are placed in order. (i.e.) in sample 8, 3, 12, 6 7, 4 the first order statistic is 3. The second-order statistic is the next least value.

A co-occurrence matrix is a matrix that is stated above an image for the diffusion of co-occurring pixel values at a given balance value. The offset value is a position provider that can be applied to any pixel in the image for over an instance.

2.6 SURVEY ON VARIOUS FEATURE SELECTION METHODS

Feature Selection is the process where the features are selected automatically or manually and further contribute to the prediction variable or the prediction. The irrelevant features in the data decrease the accuracy.

2.6.1 Discussions on Various Feature Selection Methods

Table 2.5 Literal works on Feature Selection based scheme

Sl. no	Reference	Proposed method	Application	Limitation
1	Bharti et al.(2018)	Filter Method	Enhancement	Ignore the interaction with the classifier
2	Ignisha et al. (2019)	Wrapper Method	Combination	High risk of over-fitting
3	Kalaiselvi et al. (2019)	Embedded Method	Learning algorithm	Difficult to learn

Filtering is a technique for altering or enhancing an imag Filter an image is used to bring out certain features or remove other feature Filtering includes smoothing, sharpening and edge enhancemen Bharti et al. (2018) proposed the method of hybrid feature selection (th combination of filter method and the wrapper method). It was used to obtain minimum feature set in classifying the liver stages.

Wrapper method is the selection of a set of features as a sear issue, where different combinations are analyzed, examined and compared other combinations. A predictive method is used to assess a combinatio of features and set a value based on accuracy. In wrapper methods, th classification performance of the classifier is evaluated to select the feature Wrapper methods are usually slower than filter methods but wrapper metho give better classification performance. To overcome this problem Ignisha et al. (2019) developed a strong Memetic Wrapper method. Th method is based on the collection of the mixed whale minimization algorithm with simulated annealing.

In embedded techniques, the feature selection process is integrated with the learning machine algorithm. An algorithm selects a feature in each recursive step function of the process and further divides the sample set into subsets.

2.6.1   Inference based on the Survey of Feature Selection Methods

The various feature selection methods are already discussed in the above literature review (in Table 2.5). Moreover, for the feature selection process, some of the algorithms are developed. The algorithms are listed below.

- Genetic Algorithm

- Particle Swarm Optimization

- Sequential Forward Selection

- Sequential Backward Selection

A genetic algorithm is an imitative free cost and randomly determined process with the most effective use of a situation or resource. A Genetic Algorithm takes less prior information about the issues to be solved than other conventional methods. A genetic algorithm is a method which is used to find out the solution for both natural and unnatural optimization issues based on a natural selection process. The series of points determine an optimal solution. Genetic Algorithm provides a simple, standard, and more robust structure for feature selection.

In particle swarm optimization, simple elements, called particle move in the search space of an optimization issue. Particle swar optimization is used to solve complicated issues in pattern recognitic and image processing. Particle Swarm Optimization method is used in imag segmentation for Magnetic resonance image and this method yields to achiev better accuracy than other methods. For particle swarm optimization, settir the parameters is a challenging task. Image segmentation takes place particle swarm optimization.

A sequential algorithm is used to reduce the number of feature The feature selection method based on Sequential Forward Selection is use to estimate the prediction error. The sequential forward selection algorithm a down-up procedure which begins from an empty data set and adds tl selected features gradually by some variable. This method involves forward selection by adding features one at a time,

Sequential backward selection begins from the full data set. Aft that, for each backward step it removes the selected features gradually b some function. This method involves in backward selection by removir features one at a time until some condition is reached. Moreover, bidirectional selection method is a method that includes adding or removing feature at each step.

2.7   SURVEY ON VARIOUS CLASSIFICATION METHODS

Image classification determines the numerical properties various image features and formulates data into the group. In testing feature the feature space separations are used to classify the image features. Th description of training features plays a vital role in the classification.

2.7.1　　　Discussions on Various Classification Methods

The above mentioned classifiers are already discussed in the above literature review.

Table 2.6 Literal works on Classification based scheme

Sl. no	Reference	Proposed method	Application	Limitation
1	Ahamed shaker *et al.* (2019)	Logistic Regression	Estimation	High reliance
2	Ramana *et al.* (2011)	Naive Bayes	Conditional probability	Data scarcity
3	Esraa M *et al.* (2014)	Support Vector Machine	Classification algorithms	Several key parameters
4	Henry *et al.* (2008)	Kernel Estimation	Statistical pattern recognition	Long training time
5	Aman *et al.* (2016)	K-Nearest Neighbor	Classification and regression	Lazy learner
6	Nazmun *et al.* (2018)	Decision Tree	Big datasets	Unstable
7	Ain Najwa *et al.* (2019)	Random Forest	Classification and regression	Complexity
8	Yang yu *et al.* (2018)	Deep Learning	Multiple Surfaces	Expensive to train

Logistic regression is a statistical approach which converts a logistic function to a binary dependent variable, even under complex problems. In regression analysis, logistic regression is used to estimate the parameters. Logistic regression is a form of binary regression.

Ahamed shaker *et al.* (2019) proposed a method to estimate the probabili occurrence of chronic liver diseases. Logistic regression abilities were used estimate the probability of liver disease occurrence.

Naive Bayes classifiers are a family of classification algorithm based on Bayes' Theorem. It is not a single algorithm but a group algorithms where all of them share a general principle, i.e. the features of eac pixel classified is independent of each other. The Naive Bayesian classifier based on Bayes' theorem with independence presumption between estimator Bayes theorem is used for calculating the conditional probability. Naiv Bayes classifier assumes the value of a predictor and it is independent of tl values of other predictors. This assumption is called conditional independenc (Ramana *et al.* (2011).

A support vector machine is a supervised machine learnir approach that uses classification algorithms between two grou classifications. Support vector machine is a supervised learning tool th analyzes the data set and recognizes the patterns. Esraa, M *et al.* (201< proposed the method, Support vector machine used for classifying the chron liver disease using datasets with different features combinations such a aspartate aminotransferase, glutamic pyruvic transaminase and Alkalir Phosphates. Evaluating the performance of a support vector machine classifi< is based on accuracy, sensitivity, and specificity.

The use of kernel density estimates in distinguishes analysis. Th kernel density estimates in statistical pattern recognition. The kernel density estimated correctly by selecting the scale of smoothing. The classification ru of kernel density estimation (Henry *et al.* (2008)) was applied to discrimina normal and cirrhosis cases.

The k-nearest neighbors algorithm is a supervised machine learning algorithm which is used to solve both classification and regression problems. It is easy to implement and understand. K-nearest neighbor based methods slow down the process, when the size of the data is in the growing period. The K-fold hybrid analysis method is used to assess the performance of k-nearest neighbor classifiers. Aman *et al.* (2016) observed that KNN based methods were more powerful than all other classifiers in terms of overall accuracy as well as classification performance. Moreover, KNN with correlation distance metric and nearest rule-based machine learning methods have improved as the best detective method with the highest accuracy.

A decision tree is a flowchart algorithm in which each internal node delineates as a test on an attribute. Each branch delineates the outcome of the test. Each leaf delineates a class. Moreover, a decision tree is used because it provides the more accuracy than other classification algorithms. The big datasets are easily classified by the decision tree and are easy to understand by the human. The structure of the Decision tree is like a tree structure. Decision tree is made up of a root, leaf nodes and internal nodes. Several decision tree techniques were used in this method (Nazmun *et al.* (2018)). They were namely Random Forest, Random tree, Decision Stump, and Hoeffding. Their performance was analyzed using Accuracy and Run time.

Random forests are combined learning method for classification, regression and other operations that operate by constructing a multi-level of decision trees at training time. The Random forest creates a family of methods that consist of forming an ensemble. It is a method to develop a random sample set of data to form a decision tree. It is one of the most powerful algorithms as it is highly capable of performing both classification and regression. Ain Najwa *et al.* (2019) proposed a method. Multiple decision trees were produced. Based on a majority vote, the best decision tree was

evaluated. The different instances can be selected to form a tree. Howeve
over fitting is one of the problems in Random Forest.

Deep learning is a group of machine learning algorithms that us
multiple surfaces to extract higher-level features from the given features se
In image processing, lower layers can find edges, while higher layers can fir
the contents relevant to a human such as digits or letters or faces. A dee
learning-based algorithm is used to classify the images without preprocessir
through learning from a big feature set of images. Yang yu *et al.* (201
investigated the performance of classification features using a deep learnir
algorithm and pre-sampled using multiple set of images to find out live
fibrosis and also compared against all other non-deep learning-base
algorithms like artificial neural networks, support vector machines ar
random forests. An automated feature classification was achieved by using
convey learning based deep learning system.

2.7.3 Inference based on the Survey of Classification Methods

The liver texture analysis method is used to extract the relevar
features for better classification. This survey (in Table 2.6) focuses on textur
methods applied to computed tomography images. Some of them are liste
below.

- Neural Network

- Minimum Distance

- Multi Level Neural Network

Neural networks are interlinked with the collection of nodes calle
neurons or perceptrons. Every neuron takes one bit of the input data, usuall
one pixel of the image, and performs a simple computation, called a

activation function for generating a result. Each neuron has a number weight that makes a difference in the result. There are several types of neural network. They are feed-forward neural network, radial Basis Function Neural Network, multilayer perceptron, recurrent neural network, modular neural network, sequence-to-sequence models and convolutional neural network.

Minimum Distance is the distance between two array values. It is the number of indices between the two values. Minimum distance occurs between any pair of equal parts in the array. The minimum distance classifier is used to classify the unknown image to classes. It minimizes the distance between the image and the class in multi-feature extent. The distance is defined as an index of same so that the minimum distance is uniform to the highest similarity.

Neural network consists of multi-layer called multiple level neural networks. A multilayer perceptron is a group of feed forward artificial neural network. A multilayer perceptron consists of more than three layers of nodes namely input layer, hidden layer and output layer. Except for the input layer, remaining layer has a neuron that employs a nonlinear activation function. A convolutional neural network is used in image processing. Some of the networks like recurrent neural networks, deep networks and deep belief systems are the examples of multi-layer neural network.

Moreover, the filtering process used to filter the detected disease increased computational complexity due to the wide spreading of disease among various diseases. However, these problems can be solved effectively through employing ultrasound-based scheme described in the prior works for monitoring the disease regularly using the measures feedback obtained from the US features.

Moreover, after evaluating with the metrics such as accuracy, sensitivity and Specificity, ultrasound-based scheme exhibited more satisfactory performance on varying the number of feature sets as well as through combining the above mentioned technique. This goodness is because the ultrasound based approach due to its natural characteristic captures all the attention of other detection mechanisms. None of the aforementioned schemes doesn't use the inexpensive cost to find out the stages of CLD disease.

2.8   GAP IDENTIFICATION

Some of the research gaps were identified with a detailed study of the literal works and they are as follows:

- Edge portions should be identified using multiple detection and classification of chronic liver disease. The remaining portion in the features set must be fully utilized for detection and classification schemes as far as possible to quickly detect the affected portion and also possible to achieve better detection rate and overall accuracy.

- An ensemble learning method should be developed to detect the chronic liver disease from the features set after training the features. Using this proposed method, the features are compared with more number of classifiers that can improve the performance based on accuracy.

- In most of the conventional methods, collection of the feature set and data have enhanced false detection and classification of chronic liver disease. Thus, an extreme learning machine based approach due to its classification performance can develop a recursive feature elimination scheme for detecting and classifying of chronic liver disease.

2.9   SUMMARY

A detailed study was done on **detection and classification methods of chronic liver disease on different features**. The study exposed different methods used in the feature classification of chronic liver disease and analyzed their merits and demerits. Moreover, ensemble learning machine and Hough histogram oriented gradient based feature extraction method, extreme learning machine and recursive feature elimination based feature selection method as well as the unsupervised learning machine and histogram equalization based feature extraction method were identified to provide much more attention and research to the upcoming proposed works.

CHAPTER 3

ENSEMBLE LEARNING MACHINE AND HOUGH HISTOGRAM ORIENTED GRADIENT BASED FEATURE EXTRACTON FOR CLASSIFICATION OF CHRONIC LIVER DISEASE

In this module, reducing the needs of the liver biopsy is done introducing a noninvasive method of classification and staging of chron liver diseases. The main objective of noninvasive method is to distributed as a practical diagnostic tool. Classification and staging CLD using noninvasive methods is based on the estimation of CLD usir Ultrasound images. The combination of ELM classifiers are used classify the different stages of chronic liver disease. A large number feature sets are used to study the experiment. The test features are 4 chronic hepatitis images, 51 compensated cirrhosis images and 4 decompensate cirrhosis images. The classification performance is bett than other classifiers using the above mentioned features. The propose method has achieved an overall performance with accuracy of 99.01% for the normal conditions, 91.45% for the chronic hepatitis disease, an 96.76% for the cirrhosis disease.

3.1   INTRODUCTION

The shape of the liver is chock like a structure and ribcag shielded. It is built up of hepatic cells that differ from millions of primar main function of the liver is to metabolism and detoxification of chemicals and drugs. It secretes bile into the intestine and helps in the process of digestion and produces protein needed for blood clotting and other functions.

Due to alcoholism, viral infections, metabolic disorders, therapeutic agents and changed immunity have grown to development of the CLD. The disease can be split into 3 stages. chronic hepatitis, compensated cirrhosis, decompensated cirrhosis. (Carey & Carey (2010), Leroy et al. (2007)). The primary stage is chronic hepatitis and is caused due to chronic inflammation of the liver.

The second stage is compensated cirrhosis. The decay of cells, inflammation and fibrous deepening of the tissue give rise to compensated cirrhosis. Compensated cirrhosis arises from the serious condition of chronic hepatic disease which is asymptomatic and hence remains unknown. (Kasper et al. (2008)).

The third stage is decompensated cirrhosis and it is the advanced stage with a severe condition which frequently ends in death. The symptoms of decompensated cirrhosis disease are ascites, jaundice, gastro intestinal bleeding, thrombocytopenia and hepatic encephalopathy. The final stage of this disease is death or Hepatocellular carcinoma (Zheng et al. (2003)).

Liver biopsy is the reference standard method for the classification and staging of CLD (Bourliere et al. (2008), Denzer et al. (2009), Castera et al. (2010)). The method allows some hurdles such as pain after liver biopsy. The problems are pneumo- thorax, bleeding, puncture of the biliary tree and rarely death due to over bleeding. Liver biopsy is avoided in the first stage itself. For the above circumstances noninvasive methods are used as a secondary for liver biopsy. From the literature review, noninvasive methods give similar performance as that of liver biopsy. (Gaia et al. (1997), Schuppan Detlef & Nezam (2008)).

Fibro test, fibro meter, transient elastography (US-base technology), hepascore and aspartate platelet ratio index are th noninvasive methods for determining condition of the liver. Fibro test used to estimate the fibrosis and inflammatory function of liver. Six serum markers α2-macroglobulin, haptoglobulin, bilirubin, gamma Glutamyl tran peptidase, Apo lipoprotein and alanine transferase are the tests included i fibro test (Cales et al. (2005), Zwiebel (1995)). Fibro test allows som unfavorable condition hence it is not preferred in most of the hospitals. Henc some classical form of classification method can be used as earlier fc identifying the healthy condition with some pathologic conditions.

3.2 EXISTING SYSTEM AND PROBLEM FORMULATION

The CBC method was used to distinguish between the healthy an non healthy conditions. If the condition is not healthy, the results wer divided into three stages as shown in figure 3.1 (Ricardo et al. (2013)). Th features were ultrasound features. The features have been extracted from Cc occurrence matrix. The decomposition was performed using wavel transform. Four classifiers have been used to classify chronic liver diseas The classifiers used are kNN, Bayes, Parzen and SVM.

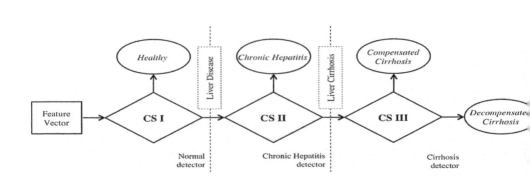

Figure 3.1 CBC Based Classification of Chronic Liver Disease

Validation of the CBC method was performed with 30 chronic hepatitis images, 36 compensated cirrhosis images, and 36 decompensate cirrhosis images. The CBC method performed better results than any other classifier method. The CBC method yields an overall classification performance with an accuracy of 98.67% for the normal condition, 87.45% for the chronic hepatitis disease, and 95.71% for the cirrhosis disease.

3.2.1 Drawbacks

- Less number of feature models

- Difficult to detect the edge portion

- Non alcoholic fatty liver disorders were not considered

- Hepatocellular carcinoma were not included

- Non minimization of false-negative rates

3.3 PROPOSED SYSTEM

Hough transform is based on the vector line of the image. The vector image line is based on the θ value of the features. It is process of a color alignment. HOG descriptor is a region developing method used to identify the region represented in the form of lines from the boundary of the region. HHOG is developed in the proposed method for the extraction of features. Ultrasound imaging is used to capture the image of liver. The image obtained from ultrasound technique is further subjected to a feature extraction process. These ultrasound features are used for the classification and Staging of CLD and also compared with clinical and laboratory characteristics of liver. These US features have more advantages in combination method than in the single method. The combination methods shall include laboratory and clinical features. The ultrasound methods are non ionizing radiation and noninvasive in nature, making US device accessible to all hospitals and easier to classify (Sebastiani et al. (2006), Castera *et al.* (2009)). This US features are used for the analysis of appearance, surface morphology and bouncing a echo of the liver.

The HHOG features are used to distinguish between norm condition and the abnormal conditions. The abnormal conditions are named Chronic Hepatitis, Compensated cirrhosis and Decompensated cirrhosis. CLD diagnosis is made in a medical centre using US images, clinical and laboratory findings. The combination of all these results provides the complete diagnosis of CLD with the experience of the medical expert. The features of HHOG reduce the contrasting diagnosis and lead to a better diagnosis. K Nearest Neighbor, Multi Support Vector Machine, Gaussian Mixture Models and Hidden Markov Model are used instead of Bayes and Parzen. The classification performance of each classifier is determined by LOOCV method. An outline of the proposed noninvasive method of classification and staging of chronic liver diseases is depicted in Figure 3.2

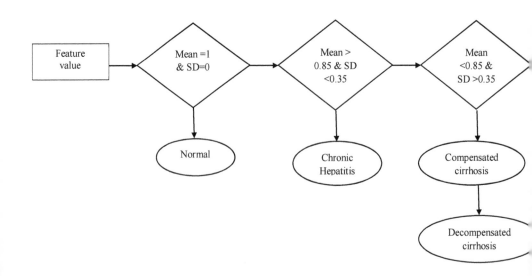

Figure 3.2 ELM Based Classification of Chronic Liver Disease

3.3.1 Images of Liver

In US images, the appearance of normal liver is in the form of homogeneous stopping by bile ducts, blood vessels and hepatic ligaments. For chronic hepatitis, it is a chance to see the repeated hepatic inflammation. In the case of Compensated cirrhosis, the normal appearance of the liver is changed to heterogeneous. Decompensated cirrhosis exhibits similar types of compensated cirrhosis, and furthermore, the shape of liver becomes non uniform. Figure 3.3 shows the images of the liver.

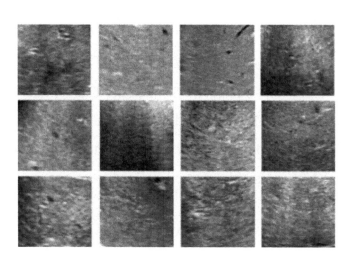

Figure 3.3 Images of Liver

3.3.2 Feature Extraction and Selection

The HHOG method is used to highlight normal liver condition from other liver abnormalities with help of mean and standard deviation values. The normal condition can be found out with mean of 1 and standard deviation of 0. In order to find the pathological condition, the mean value is below 1 and the standard deviation is above 0. In order to detect chronic hepatic disease, the mean value is kept above 0.85 and the standard deviation is kept below 0.35. For finding of compensated cirrhosis, the mean value is below

0.85 and standard deviation is above 0.35. In the most critical last stag
compensated cirrhosis is converted into decompensated cirrhosis. Hepat
Carcinoma is the last stage leading to death. Youden's index is used to sele
the classifier by considering the region of classifier. The statistics fro
Youden's J (also named Youden's index) are one statistic with a dichotomo
diagnostic test performance. Infirmity is its generalization into the conditio
of various groups and tests the probability of an informed decision. Argmax
the function that efficiently computes the argument of maximum for vecto
and matrices.

$$k), \quad k))$$ (3.

From the above equation, k represents the classifier with observe
feature set. K indicates the four classifier used in the classification proces
They are KNN, MSVM, HMM and GMM. The classifier is identified with
parameter Θ (k) and some of the features selected can be considered as f (
and hence the Youden's index is well-defined as:

$$J(k \quad k), \quad k)) \qquad ns(k, \theta(k), \quad k)) \qquad c(k, \theta(k), \quad k)) \qquad (3.$$

The KNN classifier is categorized by the lowest Euclidean distanc
criterion in the feature space according to the common of neighbours.
general the multi class SVM targets at resulting a decision plane which has
maximum. The Multi-SVM finds out a hyper plane in the new space. Th
support vector is used to divide the two features by the boundary set. Th
process can be done with the kernel function. Sens, Spec represen
sensistivity and Specificity respectively.

The HMM algorithm works on the principle of hidden states an
state transition probabilities generating the perceived symbol. HMM is use
to identify the minimum requirement. The HMM graph is shown from th

maximum point to the minimum point. Chronic liver disease is categorized by using the Gaussian Mixture Model. The mixture density function is denoted as the sum of Gaussian kernels.

$$z) \quad \sum \quad \frac{\quad\quad}{\pi)-\{\sum i-} \quad - \quad \mu)\Sigma \quad \mu) \tag{3.3}$$

From the above equation, z is a RGB color image. The Gaussian function is evaluated by a weight scalar w_i. Mean vector μ_i and diagonal covariance matrix Σ_i. Therefore, introduction of a new concept of Liver Probability Map is expressed in the following formula. The proposed method may produce a Liver Probability Map of complete image obtained by the formula of each pixel by pixel.

$$\text{LPM}(Z) = \frac{z)}{z)} \tag{3.4}$$

The application is involved with clinical and the image features extracted from multimodal sources. The process of extracting the useful information and removing unwanted information from the image is called future descriptor.

3.3.3 US Features

U.S.-based features are used in the selection of features. In HHOG, the distribution is based on histograms and the gradient direction is followed by the gradient orientation. Orientation is an angular θ based and color is based on the intensity of RGB image. The x and y derivatives represent the gradient where orientation is based on angular line. Color plays a vital role in the extraction process of features.

In HHOG process, the features are determined on a 128×128 patch scales are determined at various locations of the image. The only similarity that the patches determined have a stable aspect ratio. In the HHO descriptor, the determination of horizontal and vertical gradient lines is the first process and the second process is the determination of the gradie histogram. This process can be simply attained by removing unwanted porti in the image. The X indicates the vertical line of gradients, while the indicates the horizontal line of gradients. The sharp change in intensi increases the magnitude of gradient. If there is no change in the magnitud then consider the region to be smooth. The image is divided into 8X8 cell and for each cell the histogram of gradients is determined. The 8X8 ima patch has a value of 192 pixels. The pixel-based image patch has magnitud and direction that generates= 128 numbers.

3.4   CLINICAL AND LABORATORY FEATURES

Clinical and laboratory tests play a vital role in the detection liver disease. Hepatic insufficiency, liver inflammation, necrosis, fibrosi hyperdynamic circulation and portal hypertension are the clinical featur of CLD. Albumin, total bilirubin, prothrombin time and port systemi encephalopathy are the hepatic insufficiency suggested by pugh score the child. The time of the prothrombin is expressed as INR. Based enzymes such as aspartate aminotransferase, Gamma glutamyl transferas alanine transaminase and lactate dehydrogenase are used to determine th Liver inflammation, fibrosis, necrosis and histology of the liver. Th laboratory test may identify the changes in the liver. Differences of AS and ALT show the leakage of damaged hepatic cells.

The albumin and International Normalized Ratio reports ma reduce the growth of hepatic cells. If the discharge of free water throug the kidneys fails to function properly, there is a sodium imbalance. Th and renal excretory functions. The LDH with increased level shows neoplasms with hepatic function leading a way for hepatocellular injury.

The patients with CLD have clinical data such as age, gender, the origination of the disease and the existing problems. The originations of CLD are long term usage of alcohol, viral hepatitis and nonalcoholic fatty liver disease. The symptoms of Nonalcoholic fatty liver disease are obesity, high cholesterol and high blood pressure. Based on the etiological factors, the patient can be categorized as no disease, alcohol, hepatitis virus and other factors.

To identify the temporality rate in CLD, the child pugh score is used as a tool. Characteristics of child pugh score are ascites, GI bleeding, encephalopathy, prothrombin time and serum albumin and bilirubin levels. The acquired values are denoted as value 1, value 2, and value 3. By comparing the CLD prognosis rate with the above-mentioned calculated values, the best, moderate, and worse prognosis is observed.

Problems such as encephalopathy, GI bleeding, ascites, tumours and infections are clinically evaluated on the basis of presence or absence. The above stated problems have marked the seriousness of changes in CLD stages (i.e. chronic hepatitis to compensated cirrhosis or compensated cirrhosis to decompensated cirrhosis). Ascites is a general problem with cirrhosis. It is an accumulation of fluid in the peritoneal cavity. It has an insufficient prognostic cause. The symptoms of ascites include portal hypertension, and the rennin angiotensin aldosterone leading a way to increase the hydrostatic pressure in hepatic cells

The presence of GI bleeding involves peptic ulcers, esophageal varices and mucosal congestion. Due to the presence of any one of the characteristics such as melena, hematemesis, hematochezia, or the combination of characteristics shows the presence of GI bleeding from th esophageal varices and mucosal congestion. Growth of hepatocellul carcinoma may further increase the severity of the disease at any stage.

3.5   CLASSIFICATION OF CLD

The classification is used to categorize the different stages disease. Among three classifiers such as KNN, multi-SVM, and HMM one classifier is selected for each classification.

3.6   SIMULATION RESULTS AND ANALYSIS

The results of the proposed method are set out in this section, whic is achieved using actual data. The results are obtained by using MATLA Among the three classifiers such as KNN, multi-SVM and HMM, on classifier is selected for each classification that is based on minimum error.

3.6.1   Input Image

The image used to classify the CLD is determined by 45.7×45.7mm image. The image is selected in different sizes. The inp image for the proposed method is shown in Figure 3.4.

3.6.2   GIST Points

The image is converted into patches by using preprocessor. Patche observed on scales are determined at different locations of the image. Th only similarity is that the patches determined have a stable aspect ratio. Th proposed GIST points are shown in Figure 3.5.

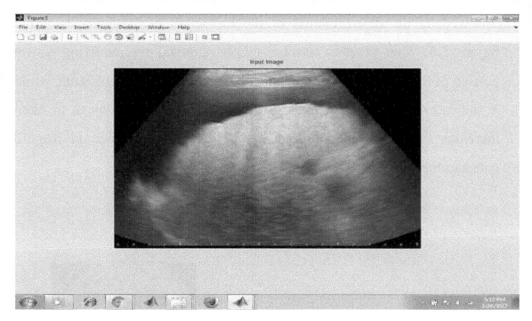

Figure 3.4 Input Image

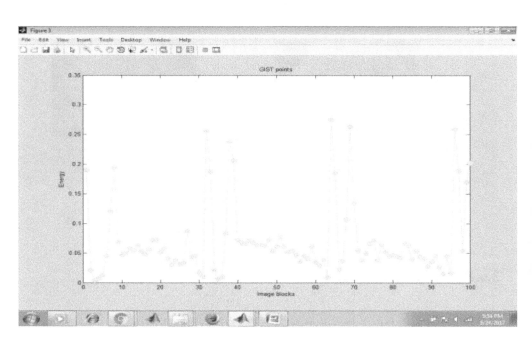

Figure 3.5 GIST Points

3.6.3   Coefficients of Feature Points

In the calculation of the coefficients of characteristics, the determination of horizontal and vertical gradient lines is the first process followed by the determination of the histogram of gradients as shown : Figure 3.6. This process can be simply attained by removing unwante portion of the image. The X indicates the vertical lines of gradients, while tt Y indicates the horizontal lines of gradients. The sharp change in intensit increases the magnitude of gradient. If there is no change in magnitud consider the region to be smooth.

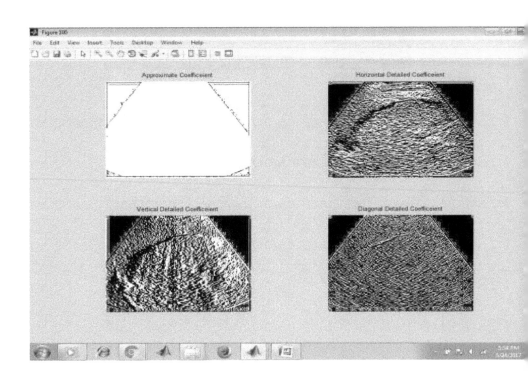

Figure 3.6 Coefficients of Feature Points

3.6.4   Detected Region of liver

The detected portion of the liver is shown in Figure 3.7. Tt detection process is divided into three categories, namely GIS Descriptors, Reconstructed Image and Detected Image.

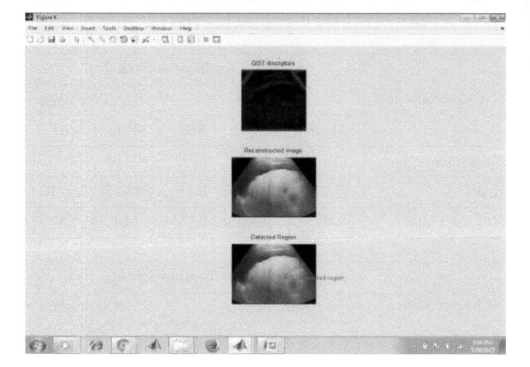

Figure 3.7 Detected Region of liver

Table 3.1 Classification Performance with Tested Features Set

Classification Step	Feature Set	Stage	Detection Rate (%)	Overall Accuracy (%)	Youden's Index	Classifier
			Classification Performance			
I	A	N	98.72	99.01	0.977	Proposed K=1,d=1,z=1
		P	99.8			
	B	N	98.61	98.6	0.985	GMM
		P	99.72			
II	A	CH	89.98	91.45	0.89	Proposed K=1,d=1,z=1
		C	90.24			
	B	CH	89.9	88.79	0.878	GMM
		C	88.46			
III	A	CC	94.99	96.76	0.93	Proposed K=1,d=1,z=1
		DC	97.99			
	B	CC	92.6	92.45	0.89	GMM
		DC	95.35			

Table 3.2 Classification Parameters of the Selected Features

Characteristics	Classification Step I					
	Normal			Pathologic		
	Mean	SD	MC	Mean	SD	MC
Glycemia	118.45	46.56	0.077	199.68	58.97	0.16
LDH	417.55	203.67	0.13	283.35	266.46	0.3'
Disease Cause	0.065	0.23	0.06	2.64	1.87	0.15

Characteristics	Classification Step II					
	Normal			Cirrhosis		
	Mean	SD	MC	Mean	SD	MC
$a_{0,1}$ (LH_1)	0.05	0.26	0.39	-0.096	0.23	0.186
$a_{1,0}$ (HL_2)	0.13	0.11	0.21	0.086	0.076	0.16
ALT	132.01	240.35	0.28	67.26	73.18	0.15
Age	53.25	17.15	0.19	62.15	13.27	0.11

Tables 3.1 and 3.2 provide an analysis of the performance of different classifiers on the basis of mean, standard deviation and mutual correlation values. For the KNN classifier, 7 different configurations are checked i.e. $K = 1, 2,....7$. The multi support vector machine polynomial trained between the degree $d = 1,2,3,4,5$ and the cost ranging c 1,10,100,500. The HMM algorithm works on the principle of hidden state and state transition probabilities that generate the perceived symbol. HMM used to identify the minimum requirement and the HMM values are indicated as $Z = 1,2,3$. The HMM is shown from the maximum point to the minimum point. For normal detector, the classifier values stated in CS I is same in both decomposition strategies. The best classification performance results are attained by setting the value as 1 for all the three classifiers. Using the above

mentioned classifiers, the detection rate for normal condition of liver is 98.72% and for pathological conditions of liver is 99.8%. The detection rate for chronic hepatitis disease is 89.98% and for cirrhosis of liver disease is 90.24% which is determined by the combined ELM classification. Ultrasound features, laboratory tests and clinical findings are used in the classification of CLD. The significance of Ultrasound features is studied by comparing the multi scheme method. 100% detection rate is achieved for normal condition of liver in both the sets. The best classification performance result for classification I is obtained using KNN classifier. In the case of chronic cirrhosis disease, the best classification performance result is achieved by the HMM classifier using the above-mentioned multimodal method.

In this study, the staging and classification of liver disease is based on the HHOG method for the extraction of features and the Combined ELM Classifiers method. The HHOG descriptors are used to detect the edge of the region in given image. The combined ELM classifiers are applied in this method to find out the chronic liver disease. The proposed ELM based classifiers for CLD are tested with a database containing multimodal data from 148 patients especially for this research. The selection of the appropriate features from different sources at each stage of classification enables optimisation. Multimodal data are collected from Government Hospital, Tirunelveli.

3.7   PERFORMANCE ANALYSIS

Performance is assessed by comparing one to all classifiers at each stage of classification. For each step of classification,one of the four classifiers is selected on the basis of a minimum error of classification.

3.7.1 Performance of Detection Rate

Detection Rate is defined as the total number patients who a[?] affected by the disease (True Positive).

A. Detection Rate of Normal Condition

Figure 3.8, the normal condition detection rate for the propose[?] method is examined with a number of features set. The Hough-HOG base[?] method is used for selecting features. The classification takes place after th[?] selection of features. By applying the concept of combined classifiers, th[?] detection rate of the proposed method is better than the current method.

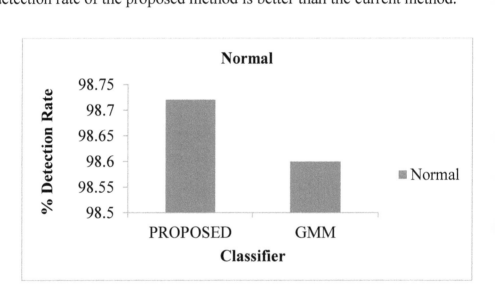

Figure 3.8 Detection Rate of Normal-Proposed Vs GMM

B. Detection Rate of Pathologic condition

Figure 3.9, the detection rate of pathologic condition for th[?] proposed method is evaluated with number of features set. For featur[?] selection, Hough-HOG based method is used. By applying the combine[?] classifiers concept, the detection rate of proposed method is better tha[?] compared to the existing method.

C.   Detection Rate of Chronic Hepatic Disease

The detection rate of chronic hepatic disease for the proposed method is examined with number of features set as shown in Figure 3.10. The Hough-HOG based method is used for selecting features. The classification takes place after the selection of features. By using the combined classifiers concept, the detection rate of proposed method is better than compared to the existing method.

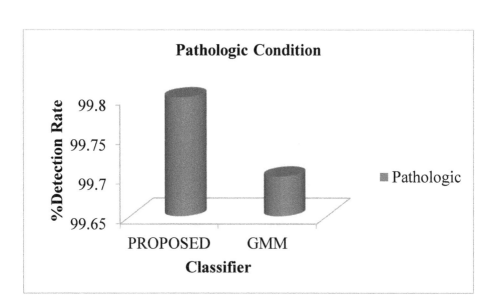

Figure 3.9 Detection Rate of Pathologic-Proposed Vs GMM

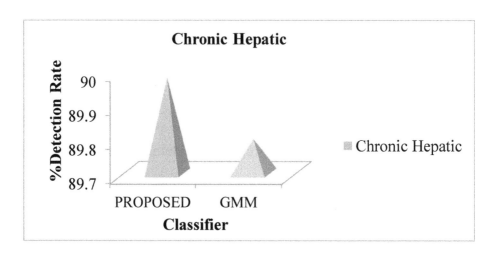

Figure 3.10 Detection Rate of Chronic Hepatic-Proposed Vs GMM

D. Detection Rate of Cirrhosis Disease

Figure 3.11, the detection rate of cirrhosis disease for the proposed method is evaluated with number of features set. For features selection Hough-HOG based method is used. By applying the combined classifier concept, the detection rate of proposed method is better than compared to the existing method.

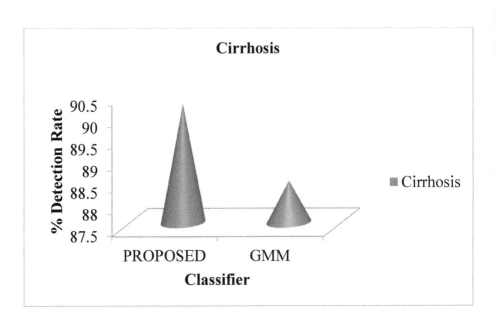

Figure 3.11 Detection Rate of Cirrhosis-Proposed Vs GMM

E. Detection Rate of Compensated Cirrhosis Disease

Figure 3.12, the detection rate of compensated cirrhosis disease for the proposed method is examined with number of features set. For feature selection, Hough-HOG based method is used. After features selection the classification takes place. By using the combined classifiers concept, the detection rate of proposed method is better than compared to the existing method.

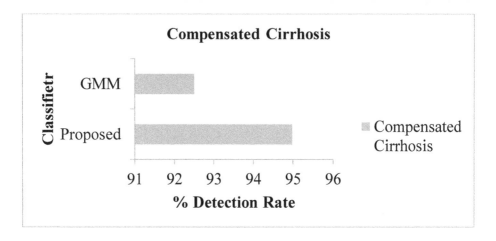

Figure 3.12 Detection Rate of CC-Proposed Vs GMM

F.   Detection Rate of Decompensated Cirrhosis Disease

Figure 3.13, the detection rate of decompensated cirrhosis disease for the proposed method is evaluated with number of features set. For features selection, Hough-HOG based method is used. By applying the combined classifiers concept, the detection rate of proposed method is better than compared to the existing method.

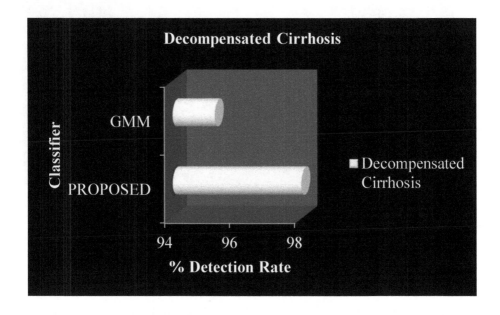

Figure 3.13 Detection Rate of DC-Proposed Vs GMM

3.7.2   Overall Performance

In order to analyze the overall performance of the proposed methc two different methods are employed on the basis of classificatic performance. In other words, the accuracy of the proposed approach analysed by varying the different number of features set. Figures 3.1 delineates that the proposed method is higher than the existing method. Fc the entire classification, proposed method has achieved better accurac compared to other method.

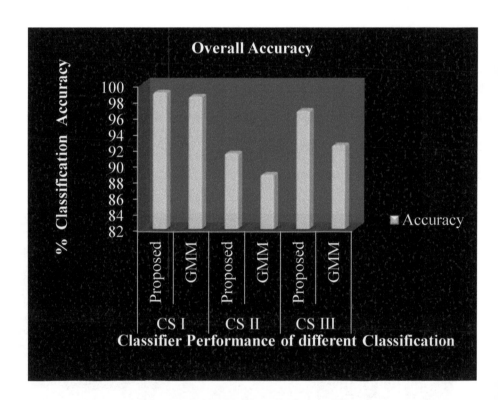

Figure 3.14 Overall Performance-Proposed Vs GMM

In proposed method it attains 99.01% for normal 91.45% for th chronic hepatitis disease and 96.72% for cirrhosis disease compared to th existing method attained only 98.6% of normal detector 87.45% for th chronic hepatitis detector and 95.71% for cirrhosis. Normally, an increase i

3.7.3 Performance of Youden's Index

In order to analyze the performance of youden's index is employed on the basis of classification performance. Figures 3.15 show that the proposed method is better than the existing method. Youden's index is used to select a classifier by considering the region of the classifier where the sensitivity and specificity of the classifier is increased when one cross validation is left out.

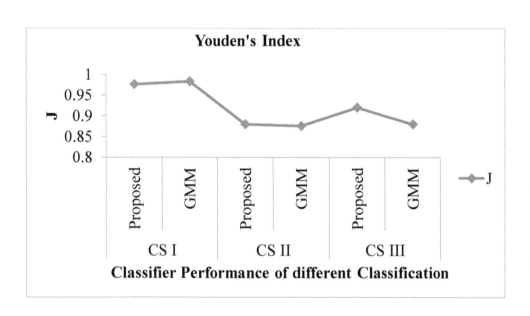

Figure 3.15 Youden's index -Proposed Vs GMM

3.7.4 Mean, Standard Deviation and Mutual Correlation for CS I

Figure 3.16, represents the results of mean, standard deviation and mutual correlation values for classification step I. By applying the combined classifiers concept and features selection method, it discriminates into two categories namely normal and pathologic.

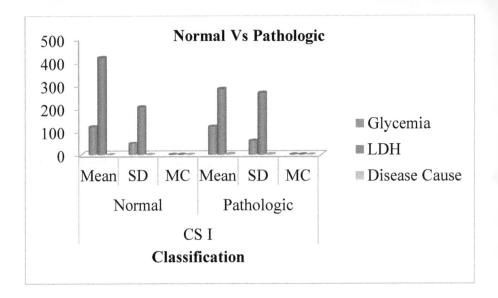

Figure 3.16 Classification Stage I

3.7.4   Mean, Standard Deviation and Mutual Correlation for CS II

Figure 3.17, represents the results of mean, standard deviation and mutual correlation values for classification step II. By applying the combined classifiers concept and features selection method, features discriminate into two categories namely chronic hepatic and cirrhosis.   The classification stage consists of chronic hepatic and cirrhosis.

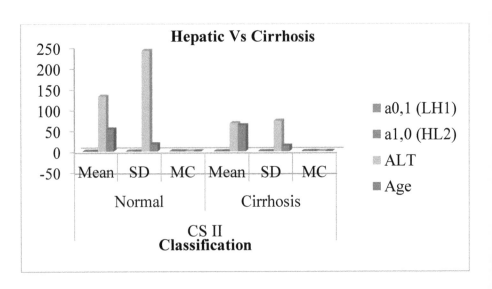

3.8   SUMMARY

In this study, the classification and staging of CLDs using noninvasive methods is proposed based on the clinical assessment of CLDs. The combined classifier mimics the differential diagnosis of CLD and performs the faster detection of the disease in clinical use. Each classification is optimized with respect to classifier and the feature set. The main objective of non-invasive methods is to be distributed as a practical diagnostic tool that can minimise liver biopsy. But this method is not completely replaced by less capability.

CHAPTER 4

EXTREME LEARNING MACHINE AND RECURSIVE FEATURE ELIMINATION BASED FEATURE SELECTION FOR CLASSIFICATION OF CHRONIC LIVER DISEASE

This module is intended to develop an ELM-RFE based selection features for the classification of CLD. The features are extracted by recursive feature elimination method in which the features are mainly involved in the detection of liver diseases. In order to identify the disease, ultrasound feature images can be used instead of CT images. Therefore this misbehavior known as the selection of ultrasound features. To classify the disease a Extreme Learning Machine (ELM) based clinical classifier is proposed and discriminates healthy from pathologic conditions. To improve the ELM performance, different types of kernels such as radial basis function (RBF) and polynomial (second and third order) are applied. The proposed layered structure identifies all the three classes of Chronic Liver diseases with highly acceptable classification accuracy of 98%, 97% and 99% for CH, C and DC respectively. The core idea of this method is to improve the performance from all other methods. Only accurate detection and classification can be carried out using this proposed method.

4.1 INTRODUCTION

Mortality and morbidity rates are high in developed countries due to large increase in chronic liver disease (CLD). Alcohol abuse and viral hepatitis are the two significant causes of CLD (Calvopina *et al.* (2019)). Asymptomatic signifies the initial stages of CLD (e.g. hepatitis or steatosis). Liver inflammation is the sign of hepatitis that can lead to liver cell destruction and damage (Andrew *et al.* (2019)). Hepatitis viruses give birth to fatal liver disease called hepatitis which is categorized into different forms based on the disease causing factors (e.g. smoking, alcohol). Hepatocellular carcinoma and cirrhosis are the crucial pathological conditions of hepatitis that increase the mortality and morbidity rate. Anatomical characterization for the chronic disease (i.e. for cirrhosis) is performed on basis of the fibrosis combined with extensive liver nodules (Hashem *et al.* (2017)). Decompensated cirhossis (a crucial form) and compensated cirrhosis (a stable form) are the two distinguishable possible cirrhosis phases (Sappagh *et al.* (2018), Ribeiro *et al.* (2012)).

In CLD staging and evaluation, the liver biopsy has played a significant role. But, the current evolutions of other advanced non-invasive alternatives have decreased the use of liver biopsy in CLD assessment. Compared to the effectiveness of biopsy, the ultrasound (US) data was considered to be the safest assessment tool in CLD staging. In (Allan *et al.* (2010)), the CLD is diagnosed using the effective features such as, surface morphological characteristics of liver parenchyma, texture characterization and echogenicity. The subjective assessment of these features has been significantly affected by the human operator. In addition, the staging and diagnosis of CLDs resulted in significant errors in the use of this factor. Essentially, the good variability can be observed with the US liver images. Hence, there is a need to improve Computer Assisted Diagnosis framework by introducing a new objective of feature extraction and classification techniques in it.

To further classify different chronic liver diseases, the ultrasoun images were analyzed by the researchers using their various propose approaches. Zhou *et al.* (2009), has used the extracted objective features c US images to assess CLD by introducing new classification procedure However, some of the well-known techniques such as, backscatterin parameters and coefficients, attenuation, wavelet transform, co-occurrenc matrix, and first-order statistics are widely adopted by most of commc features. Hepatic fibrosis has been discriminated against from US images i an experimental study in (Cao et al. (2005)). The liver parenchyma characterized from US images by computing co-occurrence informatioi entropy measures and fractal features. When a fisher linear classifier is use the overall accuracy of the classification obtained is 85.2 %.

Mojsilovic et al.(1998) characterised the spread of liver diseas from US images on the basis of the Wavelet coefficient capability. Howeve they have discriminated the conditions of cirrhotic, steatotic and normal. Th experimental study conducted has proved that wavelet based classifier ha achieved the classification accuracy in terms of fractal measures, Fourie descriptors, and co-occurence information as 69%, 82%, and 87% respectively. Based on US images, the hepatic parenchyma homogeneity measured considering the benefits of standard deviation to categorize th patients conditions as CLD (64), fatty liver (66), and normal (72 (Lee *et al.* (2006)). The significant difference between the fatty live normal, and the CLD group is $p < 0.0001$. In case of CLD group, the intensit values are distributed within ROI to obtain higher average standard deviatio values. Thereby, the liver cirrhosis and chronic hepatitis conditions ai determined on the basis of heterogeneous echo texture of CLD group

However, this was not appropriate for all types of features; therefore, they work entirely on the basis of the ROI location.

4.2 PROPOSED ELM-RFE BASED FEATURE SELECTION FOR CLASSIFICATION OF CLD

4.2.1 Extraction and Classification of Features

In proposed method, the clinical and visual are the two significant features extracted from clinical data, US image and laboratory for analysis of each patient condition.

Ultrasound Features

4.2.1.1 SIFT Feature

A local feature which can show robustness to rotation changes, translation, scale, illumination and noise is SIFT feature (Lowe *et al.* (2004)). Based on SIFT feature, the proposed method have adopted bag-of-words model for an image representation. From each training image, 30 random sampled points were used for the extraction of SIFT descriptors. Considering K-means (K=500), a visual vocabulary is produced using all of these extracted SIFT descriptors. Subsequently, the visual words are quantified by random sampling 1500 SIFT descriptors of each image. At last, the visual words containing 500-bin histogram are used to represent an image.

4.2.1.2 LBP Feature

Usually, the local gray-level structure is summarized using a measure called Local Binary Pattern (Ojala *et al.* (2002)). Along with the central pixel value, this operator takes the thresholds for the nearby pixels

Conversely, this operator takes the local neighborhood over each pix
Finally, a local image descriptor is represented using binary-coded valu
Depending on 8 pixels over the central pixel, the 8-bit codes are produced
define normally the 3×3 neighborhoods using LBP. In order to represent a
image, the LBP histogram of $256(2^8)$ bin was produced by counting t
extracted LBP codes form an image pixels.

4.2.1.3   Gabor Texture Feature

A human visual system responses can be modeled accurately usi
the Gabor filters. In extraction of texture feature, the Gabor filter base
techniques have played a significant role. Here, the implementatio
procedures of (Manjunath *et al.* (1996)) are followed. The scale sensiti
filters and orientation bank contained image are filtered to generate t
feature. In addition, the frequency domain is considered to be used
calculate the output statistical measures. In proposed method, an image
filtered using 4 orientation and 3 scaled Gabor filters. However, the 120-b
histogram feature is formed after quantizing the filtered images mean to 1
bins.

4.2.1.4   Tamura Texture Feature

Based on analysis of human visual perception textural features, t
six textural features (roughness, regularity, line likeness, directionalit
contrast and coarseness) have been proposed by (Tamura *et al.* (1978)).
the proposed method, the three basic textural features (directionality, contra
and coarseness) have been used due to the effectiveness proved in the pa
image retrieval research works. For each image, a 512 dimensional featu
vector was formed through quantizing the values obtained from the featur
evaluated based on pixel basis into a 3-dimesional histogram of 8×8×8=51
bins.

4.2.1.5 Laboratory and Clinical Features

Hepatic dysfunctional patients can be evaluated and managed well using various laboratory and clinical data rather than considering the image based features. Hence, the ten features selected from the clinical data (gender, age, Child-Pugh score, alcoholic habits, infection, gastro-intestinal bleeding, encephalopathy, ascites, tumor and disease cause) as well as the 11 features selected from the laboratory tests (lactate dehydrogenase (LDH), urea, sodium, glycemia, gamma-glutamyl transferase (gGT), Alanine Transaminase (ALT), aspartate aminotransferase (AST), creatinine, albumin, international normalized ratio (INR) and bilirubin) are applied for the determination of Hepatic dysfunctional patients.

4.2.2 Feature Selection and Classification

The most informative and appropriate feature sets can be identified with the help of feature selection technique. Hence, the classification accuracy is improved with the selection of these most appropriation feature sets. By the fact, the data size reduction can enhance the convergence speed of the algorithm as well as minimize the computational time. In different applications, the non-linear Extreme Learning Machine (ELM) when combined with recursive feature elimination (RFE) method has proven its effectiveness over all the variants.

Considering all features, the backward elimination methods based on a selection criterion removes the features from the data in an iterative manner until a termination condition is achieved. Chatterjee, S et al.(2019) stated that the selection algorithm or backward elimination technique based on weight is an alternative form of RFE. The main functionality of RFE technique is to identify the causes that reduce the margin by training the ELM classifier using whole feature set.

The basic extreme learning machine consists of a hidden singl
layer feed forward network that randomly selects the input weight in whic
the tuning process is not necessary in the case of a hidden layer. Th
expression for the output function with respect to the output weight and th
hidden layer is given in the following equation.

$$F(x) = \sum_{j=1}^{l} \alpha_j H_j(x) = H(x)\alpha$$

(4.

From Equation (4.1) the value for α ranges from $\alpha = [\alpha_1, \alpha_2, ... \alpha_l$
is the output weight among the output node and concealed layer of
concealed nodes in vector form. Then the concealed output layer in vecto
form with reference to the input is given by $H(x) = [H_1(x), H_2(x), ... H_l(x)$
and the activation function for the ELM classifier is represented in Equatic
(4.2).

$$h\alpha = t$$

(4.2

From the above equation the value for h, α and t value a
described as follows.

$$h = \begin{bmatrix} g(W_1.X_1 + B_1) & \cdots & g(W_l.X_1 + B_l) \\ \vdots & & \vdots \\ g(W_1.X_n + B_1) & \cdots & g(W_l.X_n + B_l) \end{bmatrix}_{n \times l}$$

(4.

$$\alpha = \begin{bmatrix} \alpha_1^t \\ \vdots \\ \alpha_1^t \end{bmatrix}_{l \times M}, \quad t = \begin{bmatrix} T_1^t \\ \vdots \\ T_1^t \end{bmatrix}_{l \times M}$$

The value for α is evaluated by applying the generalized form of Moore Penrose inverse matrix. Therefore, $\overset{\wedge}{\alpha} = h^+ t$ whereas $h't$ and hh' is said to be non-singular matrix when $h^+ = (h^t h)^{-1} h^t$ and $h^+ = h^t (h^{-1} h^t)$.

The condition for the data analysis is n < 1 and to enhance the system stability of the extreme learning machine the value for α is to be evaluated and it can be expressed as

$$\overset{\wedge}{\alpha} = h^t \left(\frac{I}{C} + hh^t \right)^{-1} t \qquad (4.4)$$

From the above equation, the regularized coefficient value is expressed as 'C'. Then the definition for the Multiple Kernal ELM matrix is described as $\varepsilon = hh^t$ and in terms of ith and j^{th} matrix equation is represented by $\varepsilon_{ij} = h(x_i) h(x_j) = k(x_i, x_j)$. The expression regarding the output function of ELM can be obtained by the following equation.

$$F(x) = \begin{bmatrix} k(x, x_i) \\ \vdots \\ k(x, x_n) \end{bmatrix} b \qquad (4.5)$$

From the above equation,

$$b = \left(\frac{I}{C} + \varepsilon \right)^{-1} t \qquad (4.6)$$

Therefore the category equation for an unknown sample $\overline{Y}$ is achieved in the below expression.

$$Cat \, (\overline{Y}) = Arg \, M \, (F(\overline{Y})) \qquad (4.7)$$

The ranking criterion for feature k is the square of the element of $^\alpha$,

$$J(k) = \alpha_k{}^2$$

(4.8

Training of the ELM model is performed towards all iterations the RFE in order to identify the smallest weight valued features fo elimination; therefore the accuracy of the classification is greatly improved.

In each run, a single feature is removed and the next iteration performed through inputting residual features into the ELM classifier mode Repeatedly, this feature elimination technique is carried out until all th features are eliminated. In the next stage, high importance is given to th feature that was last removed. But, this elimination method does not wo properly on a high dimensional feature vector due to increased tim consumption during feature selection process.

To tackle this hurdle, the technique of eliminating more than on feature in a single iteration is proposed. In the case of highly correlate features, more than one feature in a single iteration is removed b constructing a feature group. In a way of correlated feature group, the feature were eliminated by selecting elimination threshold value parameter at th feature elimination stage. This process is done if the predefined paramete value is found to be smaller than the number of features.

Hence, in feature selection process, the time consumption significantly reduced using this correlated feature elimination technique a shown in figure 4.1. The elimination of correlated features from the va feature set will help to identify important features. It can be concluded tha this technique is suitable for other kinds of similar topological problems.

Algorithm 1: ELM-RFE Feature Selection
Input: A set of training samples with feature dimension d;
An non-linear ELM training algorithm; T_a .
1: Initialize the list of existing features $F_{in} \leftarrow \{1,...,d\}$; the list of eliminated features $F_{out} \leftarrow \phi$;
2: *while* $F_{in} = \emptyset$ **do**
3:    Train an ELM model with the features in F_{in}.
4:    Calculate the features' ranking criteria
5:    Sort F_{in} according to descending order of the ranking criteria.
6:    if $\left| F_{in} \right| > T_a$ **then**
7:        $r = \min\left(floor\left(\left\| \frac{F_{in}}{2} \right\| \right), \left| F_{in} - T_a \right| \right)$
8:    *else*
9:        $r = 1$.
10:   **endif**
11:    $F_{removed} \leftarrow$ the last r elements in F_{in}; $F_{in} \leftarrow$ the first $|F_{in}| - r$ elements in F_{in}.
12:    $F_{out} \leftarrow [F_{removed}, F_{out}]$.
13: *end while*
Output: A ranked list of features $F_{ranked} = F_{out}$, the most important feature in the first place.

Figure 4.1 Feature Selection Technique Algorithm

4.2.3   Image Classification

For various biomedical applications, the past literal works have suggested (Ozkan *et al.* (2018), Shao *et al.* (2019)) different classification strategies. In order to classify different chronic liver diseases, a multi-class classification technique is introduced in the proposed research work. In the initial stage, the accuracy of the classification should remain higher in order to achieve accurate classification at each stage of the classification.

4.3   PROPOSED SYSTEM DIAGRAM AND EXPLANATION

The main objective of the proposed work is to develop an effective algorithm for detection and classification in US images. Initially, the extraction of features is performed to detect chronic liver disease. In addition, the selection of features is made to discriminate against healthy and pathological conditions.

In proposed method, the three diseases are classified by introducing a new layered structure of classifier (shown in Figure 4.2). In order to discriminate against healthy images from other chronic liver diseases, the 'CLR 1' (means classifier 1) has been introduced in the proposed classification strategy. On the other hand, this classifier includes two different classes namely, the positive class (contains the healthy images) and negative class (group of other diseases).

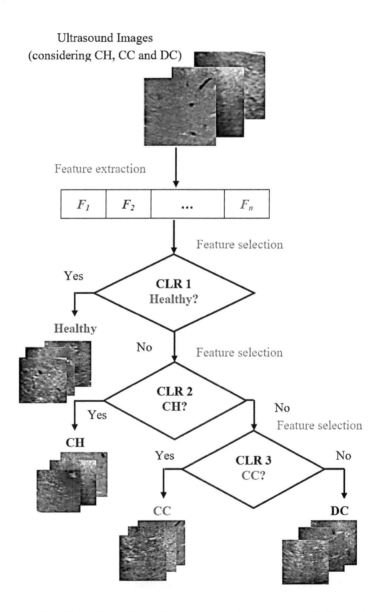

Figure 4.2 Classification Strategy using Layered Structure

Prior to the classification process, the ELM-RFE feature selection method is used to select the features that have the ability to discriminate between healthy images and all other diseases. CLR 2 (means classifier 2) is introduced in the second level to differentiate CH from CC. At last, the CC from the other misclassified images (grouped as DC) is differentiated by means of introducing a binary classifier called CLR 3 (means classifier 3).

Algorithm 4.1: Algorithm for ELM based classification using the proposed scheme

Step 1:	Feature extraction: Visual and Laboratory & Clinical Features are extracted
Step 2:	Feature selection: The feature selection is done by ELM-RFE method
Step 3:	Implementation of a single learning process and evaluating the matrix 'b' by using Equation (4.6)
Step 4:	Obtain ELM matrix using $\varepsilon_{ij} = h(x_i)\,h(x_j) = k(x_i, x_j)$
Step 5:	Evaluation of network output by using Equation (4.5)
Step 6:	Determination of sample category using Equation (4.7).

4.4 SIMULATION RESULTS AND ANALYSIS

The experimental analysis of proposed ELM-RFE based features selection and classification of chronic liver disease is done in the MATLAB platform. The performance is also determined by comparing the efficiency of conventional classifier such as SVM –Support Vector Machine, Artificial Neural Network (ANN), Naïve Bayes (NB), Decision Tree (DC) schemes with some well-known parametric measures namely, Sensitivity, Specificity and Accuracy.

A medically validated liver information containing dataset wa developed. In the proposed method, 100 patients with CLD conditions we analysed from Vien Hospital in Tamilnadu, India. Based on the results of liv biopsy, the patients diagnosed with the disease were selected. If found th patients have undergone treatment before six months or they are with oth liver disease, then these patients were eliminated. According to CLD stagin the number of patients diagnosed with CH is 30, CC is 34, and DC is 3 Further, 39 patients are affected by CLD due to virus infection (HCV=28 ar HBV=11), 32 patients due to alcoholic consumption, and 14 patients due t other causes or the combination of both ($n = 15$).

Healthy (normal) class was included in the 50 volunteers containir control group. In the same day, the US images, clinical history, and laborator tests were performed for each database sample ($n = 150$). Experiment validation includes 150 images of US liver collected from 150 patients.

Based on the ranking criterion, the most significant features wer selected using ELM-RFE feature selection algorithm; hence, the classificatic performance is improved. Classification performance indices are evaluated t determine the kernel hyper parameters and related kernel function of suppo vector machine classifier. Furthermore, the grid search based algorithm used to estimate the kernel scaling parameter, penalty parameter of so margin cost function and kernel hyper-parameters.

The three types of kernel functions namely, polynomial kernel (2n and 3rd order) and radial basis function (RBF) were preferred when selectin the kernel function. For each classifier, the classification performance indice (ACC, SP, and SN) are determined by considering each kernel functions.

When compared to the performance of 2nd and 3rd order RB kernels, the ELM classifier combined with RBF kernel has obtaine achievable results (indicated in Table 4.1). The three basic classification parameter (correct Classification Accuracy (ACC), Specificity (SP), and Sensitivity (SN)) are used to summarize the classification performance of each classifier stage.

$$SN = \frac{TP}{TP + FN} \tag{4.9}$$

$$SP = \frac{TN}{TN + FP} \tag{4.10}$$

$$ACC = \frac{TP + TN}{TP + TN + FP + FN} \tag{4.11}$$

In Equation (4.9), (4.10) and (4.11), TP (True Positive) = Positive samples classified as positive; TN (True Negative) = Negative samples classified as negative; FP (False Positive) = Negative samples classified as positive; FN (False Negative) = Positive samples classified as negative.

Table 4.1   Classification Study on Classification Performance for the ELM Classifiers with different Kernels

Kernel	CLR 1			CLR 2			CLR 3		
	Sens	Spec	Acc	Sens	Spec	Acc	Sens	Spec	Acc
Polynomial (2nd order)	96.2	97.4	96.4	97.3	98.1	97.6	97.8	97.6	97.8
Polynomial (3nd order)	97.4	98.1	97.9	98.3	98.3	98.0	98.1	98.7	98.6
Radial Basis Function	98.5	98.3	99.0	99.4	91.4	98.4	99.6	100	99.6

In proposed layered structure model, the three disease classes a
classified by decreasing gradually the number of training samples in ea
layer. Classifying the melanoma images with a higher sensitivity by the fir
layer of 'CLR 1' has ensured only minimum number of misclassified imag
in the subsequent classification stage.

Table 4.1 indicates the performance of 'CLR 2' and 'CLR ;
affected by the classification performance of first stage. ELM classifier wi
RBF kernel has been applied to classify different chronic liver disease
Furthermore, the entire dataset is divided into testing and training samples
measure the classification performance. In the entire dataset, the trainir
samples are gradually decreased from 85% to 55% to evaluate tl
classification accuracy.

Table 4.2 **Classification Performance (%) of Layer Structure usin
ELM Classifier (RBF Kernel) with ELM-RFE of Varyir
Size of Training and Testing Samples**

Classifier	Training/Testing samples (%)	Sens	Spec	Acc
CLR 1	60/40	81.48	88.63	87.32
	70/30	89.77	94.33	93.44
	80/20	98.50	98.30	99.00
	90/10	99.55	99.46	99.15
CLR 2	60/40	99.50	92.32	97.92
	70/30	99.40	91.16	97.66
	80/20	90.11	95.12	93.11
	90/10	78.70	84.12	82.41
CLR 3	60/40	99.62	88.90	99.41
	70/30	99.44	100	99.70
	80/20	87.22	92.88	91.34
	90/10	78.66	71.62	74.37

Table 4.2 indicates the classification performance of all the three classifiers achieved for each of the testing and training sets.

From Table 4.2, it can be observed that the classification performance indices are reduced with the gradual reduction of the training samples. Higher classification performance is achieved by the layered structure when dividing the entire dataset with 80% training and 20% testing samples selection. From each class, 70% of images were considered to construct the training dataset to achieve better classification of healthy (H), CH, CC and DC images. In other words, the proper balance and moderate number of testing and training samples allow for the achievement of good classification results in each stages of classification.

Table 4.3 Classification Performance (%) of Layer Structure using ELM Classifier (RBF Kernel) with and without RFE of Varying Feature Size

Classifier	No of features	ELM(RBF Kernel) with RFE			ELM(RBF Kernel) without RFE		
		Sens	Spec	Acc	Sens	Spec	Acc
CLR 1	20	96.30	97.40	97.00	76.46	90.22	81.36
	30	99.21	99.22	98.88	80.63	90.21	87.32
	40	99.46	99.30	99.70	79.62	89.68	86.90
	50	99.66	99.80	99.68	82.34	91.41	89.70
CLR 2	20	99.33	74.84	97.63	80.01	74.32	78.41
	30	99.40	91.10	97.64	83.64	71.32	80.02
	40	99.60	91.12	99.10	80.12	76.36	79.32
	50	100	96.32	99.80	86.78	81.63	82.44
CLR 3	20	96.32	96.32	97.12	62.12	87.21	76.32
	30	99.82	100	99.67	71.40	92.26	84.99
	40	99.32	99.36	99.77	70.63	92.63	86.32
	50	99.32	99.62	99.68	7.41	93.11	90.44

The layered structured classification strategies corresponding classification stage are shown in the first column of Table 4.3. For each classifier, their rankings are considered by the SVM-RFE technique (Saptarshi et al. (2019)) to determine the number of features (indicated in Table 4.3). For disease identification, the classifier is fed initially with 20, 30 40 and 50 number of selected features based on their ranking criterion.

From the entire feature set, the no. of features selected is considered to be randomly selected features if it is not applied before the SVM-RFE feature selection method for the classifier. Based on the accuracy of the classification, it is possible to evaluate the performance of the classification at each stage. Table 4.3 indicates the variation in number of features done through incrementing ten features based on their ranking criteria in SVM-RFE.

When the number of selected features has been increased, the RBF kernel has achieved classification performance (Table 4.3). Initially, in the 5 selected features, the RBF kernel included classifier has attained highly achievable result in terms of accuracy (ACC), specificity (SP), and sensitivity (SN). Table 4.3 also indicated that the SVM classifier with the RBF kernel achieved good classification performance even when the number of selected features was reduced.

Depending on linear and non-linear ELM-RFE feature selection method, the first 30 features selected with the ranking criterion are used to perform the comparative performance analysis (indicated in Table4.4). For two different classification strategies, the confusion matrices obtained are shown in Figure 4.3.

In the presence and absence of ELM-RFE feature selection strategy, the identification rate obtained for the number of test images can be observed from the confusion matrices. For linear and non-linear feature selection techniques, the initial 30 ranked features selected before classification are shown in Table 4.4 Compared to the linear ELM-RFE method, the non-linear ELM-RFE method combined with CLR 1 improved the sensitivity of healthy images (Table 4.4).

Table 4.4 **Classification Performance (%) of Layer Structure using ELM Classifier (RBF Classifier) with Linear and Non Linear RFE Technique**

	ELM with Linear ELM-RFE				ELM with Non-Linear ELM-RFE		
Classifier	No. of features	Sens	Spec	Acc	Sens	Spec	Acc
CLR 1	30	98.50	98.30	99.00	98.78	99.34	99.17
CLR 2	30	99.40	91.10	97.66	99.50	91.66	96.70
CLR 3	30	99.65	100	99.67	99.64	100	99.68

As a higher sensitivity was achieved in the first stage of the classification, the classification performance was improved in the subsequent stages. CLR 2 and CLR 3 have identified CC and DC images with an increased sensitivity of 99.49 3% and 99.63 3% respectively.

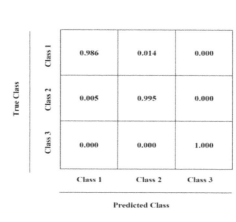

Figure 4.3 **Confusion Matrix for the Classification Performance of Healthy, CH, and CC as Classes 1, 2 and 3 Respectively**

The reported performance of the proposed classification schem can be validated from the confusion matrix as shown in Figure 4.3. Eac element of the confusion matrix represents the probability of the predictir class with respect to the ground truth or true class. From the confusion matr it has been realized that the 'CLR 1' and the 'CLR 2' in the layered mod identified healthy images (class 1 in Figure 4.3) and CH (class 2 Figure 4.3) with a high probability rate. At the final stage of the classificatio the 'CLR 3' has been able to identify all the CC and DC images efficiently.

Table 4.5 Proposed Method Comparison (%) against other Classifiers

	Classification performance indices (%)								
	Sensitivity			Specificity			Accuracy		
Classifier	H	CH	CC	H	CH	CC	H	CH	CC
SVM	93.68	95.56	95.23	95.46	93.55	97.90	95.12	94.34	96.23
ANN	94.92	94.33	95.22	96.44	92.44	97.66	95.32	93.66	97.66
NB	91.66	87.98	89.66	90.32	88.77	90.44	92.64	88.22	90.33
DT	89.66	88.63	89.66	91.66	89.63	88.63	93.62	88.66	87.66
Proposed	98.50	99.41	99.65	98.30	91.26	100	99.00	97.88	99.70

Traditional multiclass classification strategies were used compare the performance of proposed multiclass chronic liver disease classification technique. The performance result obtained is depicted Table 4.5. During training and testing stage, the same dataset is applied fo the usage of different classification strategy to classify three disease classe In multiclass skin disease classification, the proposed technique has show excellent performance than the other conventional classification technique As shown in Table 4.5, the conventional classifiers K-Nearest Neighbo (KNN) (Yu et al. (2019)), Naïve Bayes (NB) (Breiman et al. (1984)), ar decision tree has achieved less satisfactory performance compared to Support Vector Machine (SVM) (Saptarshi *et al.* (2019)) and Artificial Neural Network (ANN) (Bishop *et al.* (2006)) classifiers. Also, when compared to other traditional classifier models, the binary classifiers with ensemble classification technique have achieved satisfactory performance in the identification of multiclass chronic liver diseases.

4.4.1 Performance Analysis

A. Performance of ELM Classifier with different Kernels

In order to analyze the performance of ELM-RFE based features selection scheme three kinds of parameters are employed on the basis of features set. In other words, the efficiency of the proposed approach is analyzed by varying the accuracy, sensitivity and specificity. Figures 4.4 show the Performance for the ELM classifiers with different kernels. The proposed method is more accurate compared to the existing methods by the presence of US images. Normally, increasing the features set will reduce the accuracy. But, the proposed method attains better accuracy.

B. Performance of ELM-RFE with different Training Samples

Figure 4.5 represents the Graphical representation of performance of ELM-RFE in different samples. The performance of the system is degraded by increasing the number of training samples and decreasing the number of test samples. From Figure 4.5, it can be observed that proposed ELM-RFE method shows maximum accuracy compared to other existing methods. The reason for this fact is that, the proposed ELM-RFE method detects the chronic liver disease and classifies the disease into three categories namely healthy, chronic hepatic and cirrhosis.

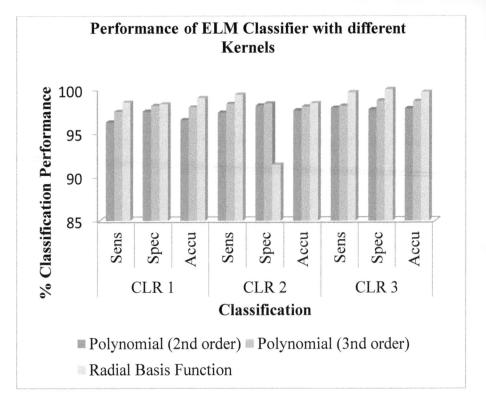

Figure 4.4 Performance of ELM Classifier with different Kernels

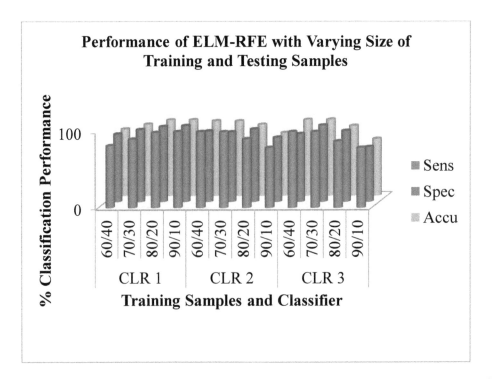

C.   **Performance between ELM with RFE and ELM without RFE**

From Figure 4.6, it can be clearly observed that the accuracy occurred in proposed method is somewhat slightly more than the other existing methods due to kernel function used in classifying the diseases. The reason for this fact is that, ELM-RFE based method is used for features selection. The performances are evaluated with different number of features. For each classifier, CLR 1 is analyzed with features like 20, 30, 40 and 50. The same procedure is applied for CLR 2 and CLR 3. Hence, the ELM with RFE is higher than ELM without RFE.

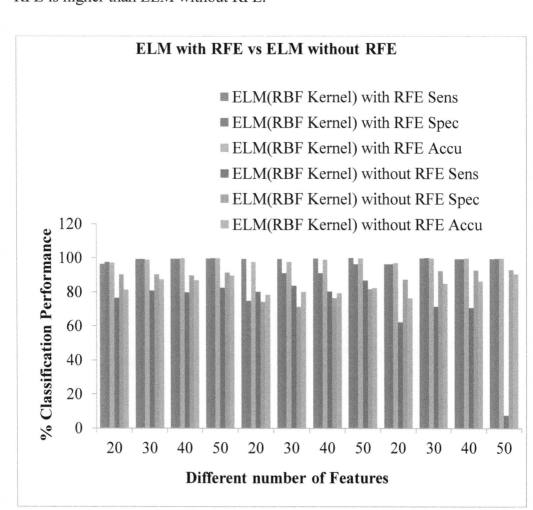

Figure 4.6   ELM with RFE and ELM without RFE Vs Classification Performance

D.   **Performance between Linear ELM-RFE and Non-Linear ELM-RFE**

The proposed ELM-RFE approach obtained very good accuracy compared to other existing approaches (indicated in Figure 4.7). ELM-RFE system efficiently detects the disease even under the 30 features set. The proposed scheme obtained the accuracy for each classifier occurred in the UI images. Hence, the ELM with non linear RFE is slightly higher than ELM with linear RFE. Compared to the linear ELM-RFE method, the non-linear ELM-RFE method combined with CLR 1 has better determined the healthy images with more sensitivity. The proposed technique has shown better performance than the other conventional classification techniques.

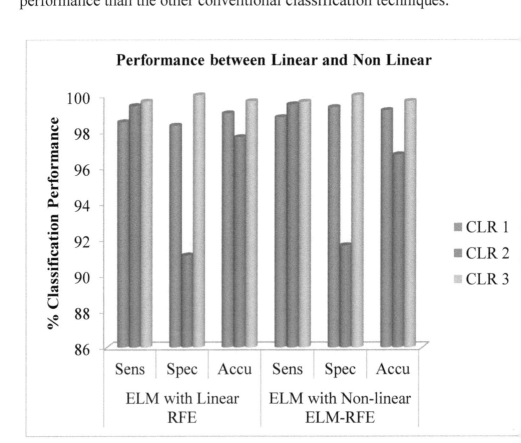

Figure 4.7 Performance between Linear and Non Linear

E. **Performance of Proposed Method against other Classifiers**

The proposed ELM-RFE method obtained very good accuracy compared to other existing methods (indicated in Figure 4.8). ELM-RFE system efficiently detects the disease using recursive features elimination method. The proposed method obtained the accuracy for each classifier occurred in the US images. The proposed technique has shown excellent performance than the other conventional classification techniques. As shown the conventional classifiers k-nearest neighbor, naïve bayes and decision tree have achieved less satisfactory performance compared to Support vector machine (SVM) and artificial neural network (ANN) classifiers.

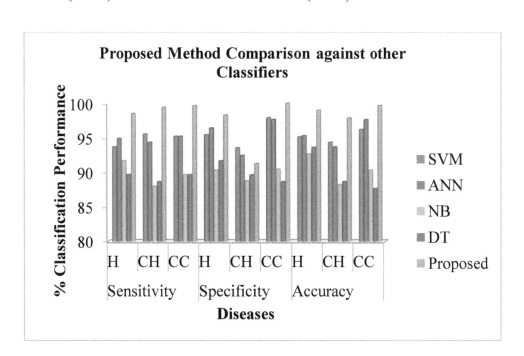

Figure 4.8 Performance of Proposed Method against other Classifiers

4.5 **SUMMARY**

In this module, to detect and classify the disease, Visual and Laboratory and Clinical Feature analysis methods have been applied for the efficient extraction of features from US images. The core idea of this method is a classification method involving recursive feature elimination (RFE) ar

Extreme Learning Machine (ELM). Using this proposed method, ELM-RF

based feature selection method prior to each stage of the layered structure

classification model has improved the multi-class classification performance

The performance of the proposed ELM-RFE method was compared with the

state-of-the-art with the proper simulation scenarios. To improve the ELM

performance, different types of kernels such as radial basis function (RBF

polynomial (second and third order) is applied From the experimental result

it was clearly observed that the proposed method attains better results in term

of accuracy, Sensitivity and specificity with considerable amount of feature

The proposed approach maintained the performance of the classification eve

though there are different training samples in the set of features of the U

images.

.

CHAPTER 5

UNSUPERVISED LEARNING MACHINE AND HISTOGRAM EQUALIZATION BASED FEATURE EXTRACTION FOR CLASSIFICATION OF CHRONIC LIVER DISEASE

This module is meant to develop a computational Intelligence based Computer Aided Diagnosis (CAD) system that helps medical Specialists to detect and diagnose the stages of CLD. The proposed method comprises the following steps are image enhancement, image segmentation and classification. The image enhancement process is performed using Histogram Equalization method. Image Segmentation is done by simple linear iterative clustering method. The classification is done by Haar Wavelet decomposition method. Initially the image of liver is pre-processed by resize and noise removal. The proposed method should be easy to perform, inexpensive, and give numerical and accurate results in real time. These methods predicted the presence of liver images with high accuracy. Finally the system is connected to the microcontroller through the Max 232 converter. The LCD will display the stages of chronic liver disease.

5.1   INTRODUCTION

In recent years, machine-learning methods such as classification made by Artificial Neural Networks (ANN) have been used as prediction, classification, and diagnosis tools (Somaya Hashem *et al.* (2017)). Machine learning methods are used in the medical field for disease detection by a invasive method for disease prediction and detection, such as fibrosis, cirrhosis, and Hepatitis C patients. When abnormal conditions have occurred the method shall clarify the results in three classes in a hierarchical basis: chronic hepatitis; 2) compensated cirrhosis; and 3) de compensated cirrhosis (Laurent *et al.* (2012)).

A computer aided diagnosis system for the liver disease is the combination of image processing and embedded system. Early Diagnosis will reduce mortality rate. Machine learning methods as non-invasive method have been used recently as an alternative method in staging of chronic liver diseases for avoiding the drawbacks of biopsy (Li Zhang *et al.* (2012)).

Liver cancer is a chronic cancer which originates in the liver. The tumor may originate elsewhere in the body but later it move towards the liver and makes severe damage to it (Smith *et al.* (1981)). In many cases it is not possible to identify the disease but symptomatically abdominal pain, and jaundice, will lead to chronic liver disease. Symptoms of liver cancer include High blood calcium levels (hypocalcaemia), Low blood sugar level (hypoglycaemia), Breast enlargement (gynecomastia), High counts of red blood cells (erythrocytosis) and High cholesterol levels. Treatment of cancer depends mainly on the size and rank of the tumor. Hepatocellular carcinoma is the most common type of liver cancer.

Annalisa *et al.* (2014) developed Left lobe liver surface method for cirrhosis detection. The left liver surface of the lobe is more applicable than the transient electrography. In patients with cirrhosis problems, Left lobe liver surface is the best non-invasive method for diagnosing cirrhosis. The method holds the best diagnostic accuracy Johan *et al.* (2016) presented a linear the gray level method which is used to estimate the gamma function. The

The method for diagnosing the liver cancer involves ultrasound images of liver. It provides accurate results. This method includes image segmentation and classification for ultrasound images, and probabilistic neural network is used to detect the tumor in the earlier stages. The automated disease identification system is not a single process. The system consists of various modules. The success rate of each and every step is highly important to ensure the overall high accurate outputs.

5.2   EXISTING SYSTEM

The block diagram of chronic liver disease is shown in figure 5.1.

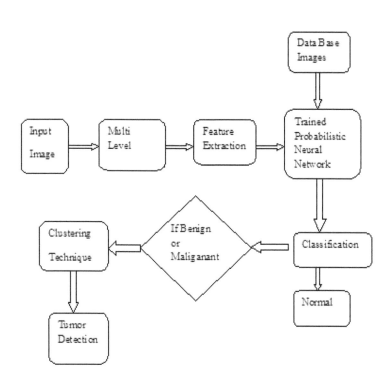

Figure 5.1 PNN based Classification of Chronic Liver Disease

The various samples of CT images were collected from Sri Swami Jnanananda Spiral C.T Scan Center Bhimavaram and also some of the other scanning centers in Bhimavaram. These images has been considered as reference images for the analysis of liver disease. The effective disease analysis depends upon the number of data base images. Wavelet transform decomposed the image into different sub band images. If the decomposition was done for more than two times it is called a multi-level wavelet transformation (Varun *et al.* (2017)). The texture features were classified using PNN classifiers. The image was converted into a reduced set of features called features vector and this conversion is called feature extraction. The reduced features represented the exact information of the input image. The features extraction was used to find the parameters like energy, contrast entropy and correlation. The Performance of the PNN classifier was determined in terms of training performance and classification accuracy.

5.2.1   Drawbacks

- For the decomposition process, most of the coefficients are not significant.

- More time taken to train the classifier.

- Low accuracy during classification.

- PNN are slower than multilayer perceptron networks for classifying new cases.

- PNN require more memory space to store the model.

5.3   PROPOSED SYSTEM

The below diagram is the block diagram of the proposed system. The US image of liver is given as an input image. The input image is further preprocessed. In preprocessing, the RGB image is converted into gray scale image and then resized. The objective of image enhancement process is to identify certain image features for the further analysis. The block diagram of proposed ULM based classification of CLD is shown in Figure 5.2.

5.3.1   Preprocessing

The aim of preprocessing is to remove unwanted distortions or enhance certain images for further processing. Here the conversion of RGB image to gray scale image is done in the preprocessing stage.

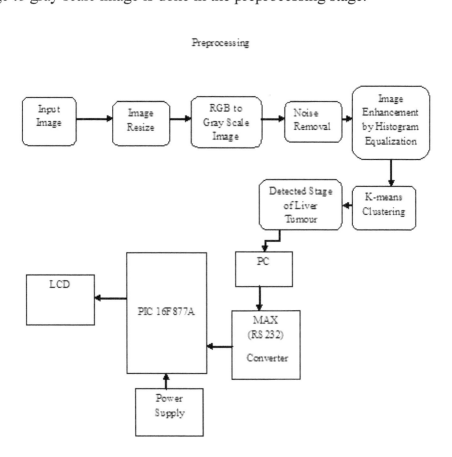

Figure 5.2 ULM based Classification of Chronic Liver Disease

5.3.2   Image Enhancement

The image enhancement method is used to point out the boundary in the image features and also used to sharpen the image features. This method is used in contrast to make the graphic display more useful for analysis. This process does not increase the inherent information content of techniques based on Contrast Limited Adaptive Histogram Equalizatic (CLAHE). This method was used for smoothing the images. This techniqu was compared using classifying performance parameters such as peak sign to noise ratio and mean square error.

In proposed method, the image enhancement is performed usir histogram equalization. Histogram Equalization is an image processir technique used to improve contrast in the images. It is done by effectivel spreading out the most frequent intensity values.

5.3.3 Image Segmentation

Image segmentation is the process of dividing an image int multiple segments (i.e. sets of pixels). It is more meaningful and easier t analyze. Image segmentation is used to find the objects and boundaries (i. lines, curves, etc.) in the images. Moreover, image segmentation is th process of giving a mark to every pixel in an image such that pixels with th same mark share similar characteristics.

In previous work, the segmentation of the image was performe using clustering algorithm (Ekong *et al.* (2011)). The key of this method is t select the threshold value. Several popular methods are used in the industr including the maximum entropy method, maximum variance method, and means clustering.

The proposed work is based on K-means clustering algorithm. is an unsupervised algorithm that is used to segment the area of interest fror the background. This method is simply to group the objects into K number c groups based on features, where K is positive integer number. Befor applying K-means algorithm, first partial enhancement is applied to th image to improve the image quality.

5.3.4   Haar Wavelet Decomposition

The Haar wavelet transform is used to determine images at various resolutions (Kamrul *et al.* (2007)). It is used to find the approximation coefficients and elaborator coefficients at various levels. The Haar transform works like a low-pass filter and a high-pass filter simultaneously. These images are then further proceeding to different levels of wavelet decomposition using different wavelets. The images are subjected to various levels (1, 2, 3 and 4) of wavelet decomposition. The synthesized image of the input image is calculated as a result. The decomposition is done to extract the certain features from the liver images. Still, these images cannot be used unless a quality process is done. In order to ensure the diagnostic accuracy of the images, the quality assessment metrics are used to obtain wavelet performance. The ultrasound liver image is decomposed into approximate, horizontal, vertical and diagonal details. The decomposition is done by N-levels. Here, 4-levels of decomposition are used. Moreover, quantization is done on the decomposed image. Quantization is done by thresholding. The wavelet function is taken based on the results of image quality parameters. In image, wavelet decomposition is performed by the number of times so that the image can be divided by twice. In each level of wavelet image decomposition, the standard image of the previous level is decomposed into four sub images The image at the top left corner obtain blurred as standard and also records the horizontal, vertical and diagonal components of the image.

5.3.5   PIC Microcontroller

PIC microcontroller is the controller that can be programmed to perform a wider range of tasks. These microcontrollers are found in a number of electronic devices such as phones, computer systems and alarm systems.

5.3.5.1 General Features

- High performance RISC CPU.

- Only 35 simple word instructions.

- All single cycle instructions except for program are two cycles.

- Operating speed: clock input (200MHz), instruction cyc (200nS).

- RAM, EEPROM, and flash memory.

- Pin out compatible.

- Deep hardware stack.

- Interrupt capability.

- Different types of addressing modes.

- Power on Reset

- Power-Up Timer

- Oscillator start-up timer.

5.3.5.2 Advantages of PIC Microcontroller

- The performance of the PIC microcontroller is very fast becaus of using RISC architecture.

- When comparing to other microcontrollers, power consumptic is very less and programming is also very easy.

- Interfacing of an analogue device is easy without any extr

5.3.6   MAX232 IC

.   The MAX232 is an electronic circuit that converts signals from a serial port to signals that are suitable for use. The MAX232 acts as a buffer driver for the processor. It accepts the standard digital logic values of 0 and 5 volts and converts them to the RS232 standard of +10 and -10 volts. It also helps to protect the processor from possible damage. The MAX232 requires 5 external 1uF capacitors. These are used by the internal charge pump to create +10 volts and -10 volts.

5.4   SIMULATION RESULTS AND ANALYSIS

The experimental analysis of proposed system is done in the MATLAB platform. The performance of proposed system is determined by obtaining the classification performance.

5.4.1   Input Image

Figure 5.3 shows the input image of the liver. The input image can be changed to gray scale image. Then it will be further processed and the stage of liver disease will be determined. The image of the liver is given as an input image. The input image is further preprocessed.

5.4.2   Gray Scale Image

Figure 5.4 shows the gray scale image of the liver. The luminance of a pixel value of a gray scale image ranges from 0 to 255. The conversion of a color image to a gray scale image is carried out by converting the RGB values (24 bit) to gray scale value (8 bit). The number of bits required to encode that image is based on the given segmentation.

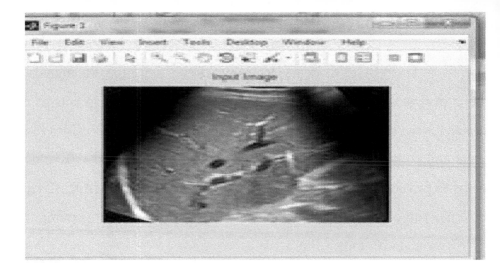

Figure 5.3 Input Image

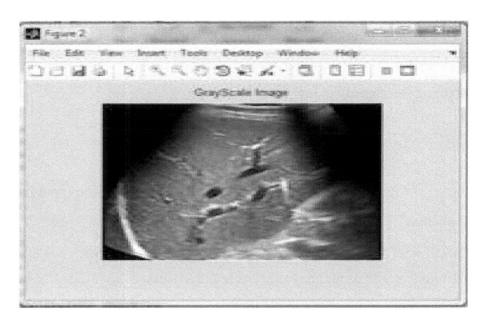

Figure 5.4 Gray Scale Image

5.4.3   Histogram Equalization

Figure 5.5 shows the Histogram equalization Image .Histogram equalization is a technique for adjusting image intensities to enhance contrast. This technique is used in image comparison processes and in the correction of nonlinear effects. Histogram based methods are very efficient compared to other image segmentation methods because they typically require only one pass through the pixels. In this technique, a histogram is computed from all of the pixels in the image. Peaks and Valleys in the histogram are used to locate the clusters in the image. Color or intensity can be used as the measure.

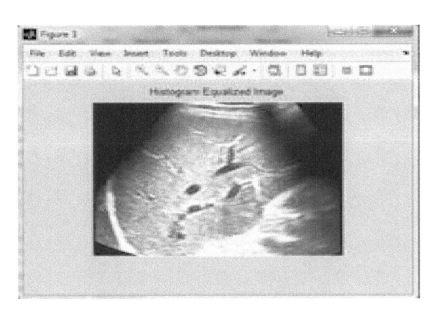

Figure 5.5 Histogram Equalization

5.4.4 LAB Image

Figure 5.6 shows the LAB image. The lab color space describes mathematically all perceivable colors in three dimensions, L for lightness and a and b for color components like green red and blue yellow. It is the process that allocates mark to an object based on its descriptors. It is the last step of image processing which use artificial intelligence.

5.4.5 K Means Clustering

K-means clustering algorithm is an unsupervised algorithm and it is used to segment the interest area from the background. But before applying K-means algorithm, first partial stretching enhancement is applied to the image for improving the quality of the image. Subtractive clustering potential value of the data points. The various cluster images are shown figure 5.7, 5.8, 5.9.

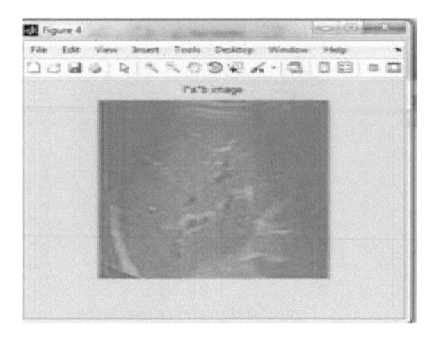

Figure 5.6 LAB image

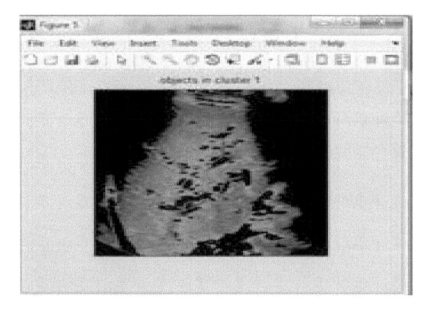

Figure 5.7 Cluster Image 1

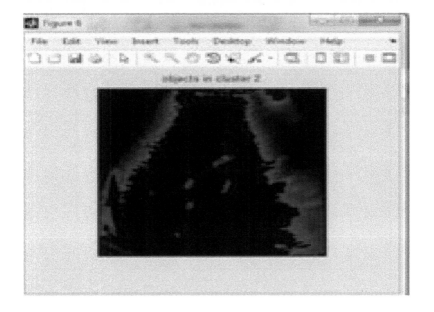

Figure 5.8 Cluster Image 2

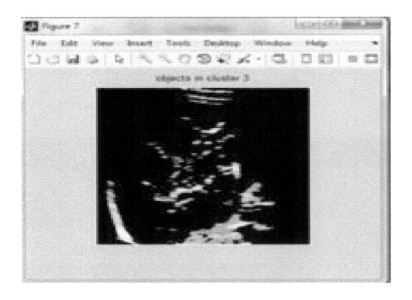

Figure 5.9 Cluster Image 3

5.4.6   CLD Detected Image

Figure 5.10 shows the output of the detected image of chronic liver disease.

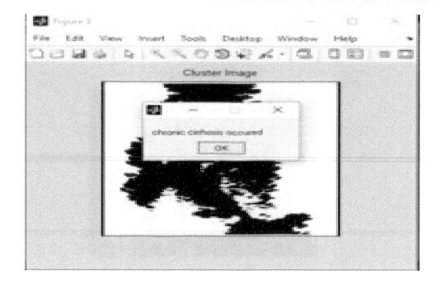

Figure 5.10 Detected CLD Image

5.4.6   LCD Output

The output of the liver disease stage will be displayed on the Liqui
Crystal Display.

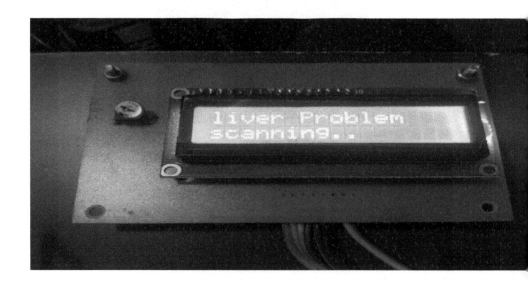

Figure 5.11 LCD Output

Table 5.1Classification Performance % against other Classifiers

Classifier	Sensitivity	Specificity	Accuracy
PSO	70.4	65.6	66.4
GA	68.9	69.7	69.6
MREG	69	69.1	69.1
ADT	73	65	66.3
ADT*	7	99	84.4
Proposed	90.23	98.10	96.4

Table 5.1 states the accuracy, sensitivity and specificity of the proposed models for finding out the CLD on the test set. The machine learning algorithms predicted CLD with accuracy between 66.4% and 84.4% (Somaya *et al.* (2017)). ADT model achieved the highest accuracy of 84.4%. The D Tree model achieved highest sensitivity of 73% and specificity of 65% but the accuracy fallen down to 66.3% while it was 84.4% using zero cut-off frequency. The ADT* model obtained the highest specificity of 99% but sensitivity got down to 7%

In proposed method, the classification performance achieved the accuracy of 96.4% and also obtained 90.23% sensitivity as well as 98.10% specificity. Comparing to other methods, proposed method attained good accuracy, sensitivity and specificity.

5.5 PERFORMANCE ANALYSIS

5.5.1 Accuracy

The classification performance achieved the accuracy of 96.4%. The proposed method accuracy is higher than all other classifiers as shown in Figure 5.12.

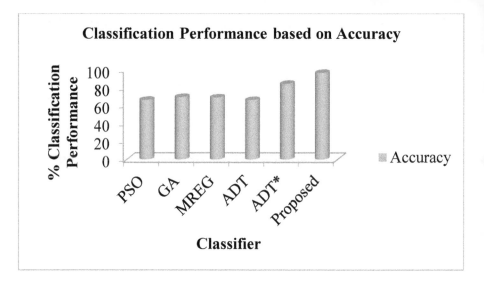

Figure 5.12 Accuracy-Proposed Method Vs other Classifiers

5.5.2   Sensitivity

Figure 5.13 shows the classification performance is based on sensitivity. The proposed method attained 90.23% of sensitivity. Compared to all other classifiers, the proposed scheme has achieved the highest sensitivity

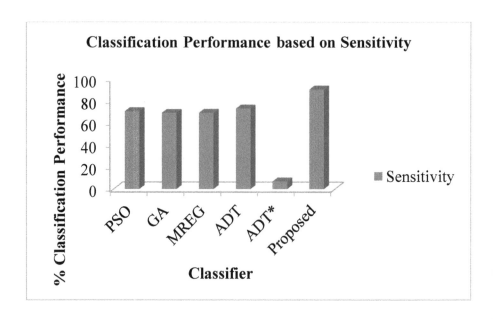

Figure 5.13 Sensitivity-Proposed Method Vs other Classifiers

5.5.3   Specificity

The classification performance based on sensitivity is shown in Figure 5.14. In proposed method 98.10% of specificity was attained. Compared to all other classifiers, the proposed scheme achieved the highest specificity. The Particle swarm optimization obtained the least specificity. From the figure, it is observed that alternating decision tree method achieved the highest specificity, but this method attained only 7% of sensitivity.

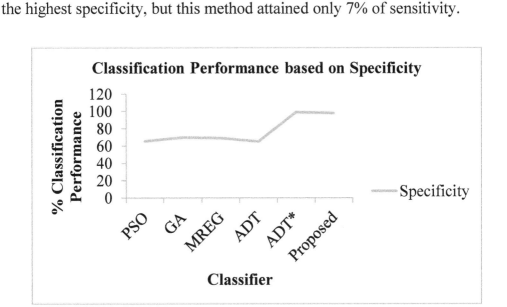

. **Figure 5.13 Specificity-Proposed Method Vs other Classifiers**

5.6   SUMMARY

In this module, to detect and to classify the chronic liver disease a new unsupervised learning machine and histogram equalization based feature extraction was introduced. Histogram equalization technique was developed in proposed scheme to detect and to identify diseases from the features of ultrasound images. The existing approaches extract the image features using wavelet transform. In that scenario sometimes the selected useful features may get blurred. At that situation the multi level wavelet transform approach can be used to select the image features and also detect the diseases using the multi level wavelet decomposition schemes. The decomposition takes place no of times and so it is called multi level process. Hence, the propose method was selected for extracting the image features very efficiently ar also segments the affected portion in the image features through k mean clustering. The selected image features was used to classify the chronic live disease with the help of morphological Haar wavelet decomposition proces The performance of the proposed scheme was compared to proper simulatic scenarios. From the experimental results it was clearly observed that th proposed scheme attains better results in terms of accuracy, sensitivity, ar specificity with considerable number of features set. The proposed approac maintained the classification performance of the chronic liver disease in th ultrasound images.

5.6 COMPARISON OF PROPOSED CLASSIFIERS

The below figure 5.14 plots the differences between the majc classifiers that have been taken for study. The combined Ensemble Learnir Machine classifier is compared with the kernel extreme learning machir classifier as shown in table 5.2. The kernel extreme learning machir classifier shows better visualization accuracy of healthy liver and the accurac seems to be the highest for all the stages of CLD.

Table 5.2 Comparison of Proposed Classifiers

S.No	Classifiers	Disease	Accuracy
1	Proposed 1		99
2	Proposed 2	H	99
3	Proposed 1		91.45
4	Proposed 2	CH	97.88
5	Proposed 1		96.76
6	Proposed 2	CC	99.70

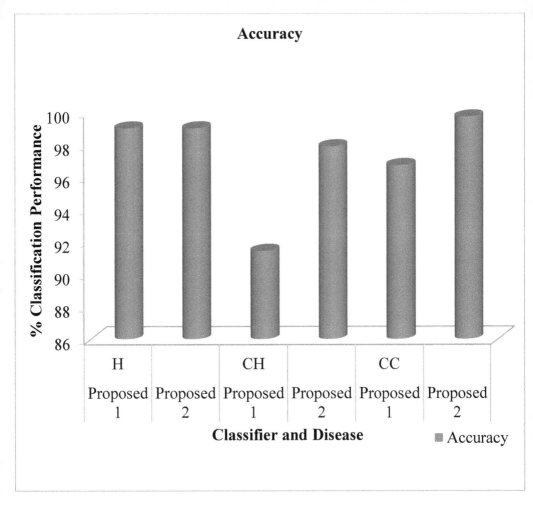

Figure 5.14 Comparison of Proposed Classifiers

H-Healthy, CH – Chronic Hepatic, and CC-Compensated Cirrhosis

CHAPTER 6

SUMMARY AND CONCLUSION

Fast-growing computer-aided diagnostics are the most widely use technologies for medical imaging. Furthermore, due to a lack of infrastructure and climatic conditions, research work is still in developing in this area. Ther are a huge number of people who have different diseases in their bodie Diseases should be diagnosis properly and further proper treatment is don However, automated diagnostics do not require any support from medical radiologists for the detection of CLD diseases. Hence, there is a great chanc of getting difficulties in finding the diseases for the medical experts. Th challenges include developing an efficient learning machine based mechanism for finding the diseases with good accuracy as well as fast performance an classification of diseases. To achieve the proposed objectives, the mo important contributions pointed by us are as follows:

As a first contribution, overall performance in detecting the chroni liver disease is improved by introducing a new ensemble learning machir and Hough histogram oriented gradient-based feature extraction fc classification of chronic liver disease. Detection of CLD in the edges of th region is the main goal of proposed mechanism. Hence, multiple detectio schemes are created and allowed them for detecting the presence of CLD a quickly as possible. Also, a detection rate of CLD is obtained further t improve the classification performance. Notably, these multi detectio schemes are better balanced and shared using the proposed mechanism thereby, ensuring the quick CLD detection. To improve the overall accuracy and minimizing the need of liver biopsy, the entire liver image from ultrasound features are selected by the proposed mechanism for the classification of chronic liver disease. In the proposed mechanism, each classification stage highly optimizes with respect to classifier and features set by avoiding the inaccurate classification and drastically increasing the computer-aided diagnosis in all hospitals.

In the second contribution, a mechanism called an extreme learning machine and recursive features elimination based selection of features is developed to enhance the conventional detection scheme when detecting CLDs that are trying to launch a collaborative method. The selected features in conventional scheme may act as an inaccurate by showing normal behavior same as that of the pathological behavior. In order to overcome this hurdle, extreme learning machine is performed using kernel functions. Also, recursive feature elimination technique is imposed to detect the CLD disease and identifying them from other diseases. However, our new proposed scheme is initiated with the following situation: the image features are selected by recursive feature elimination and further determined with radial bias function using kernel. The existing system determines the classification performance as inaccurate and then further unable to classify the different stages of CLD. Eventually the system gets failed. The proposed method inherits the conventional method principle, but incorporates a clinical classifier based on an extreme learning machine. This will help the system to identify the CLD and find out the different stages of CLD. ELM-RFE based feature selection method prior to each stage of the layered structured classification model has improved the multi-class classification performance.

A cooperative task performed in multi level wavelet transform is based on coefficients in which, the image features participate mainly in the coefficients of feature points. However, most of the coefficients are not

significant. In order to solve this problem, opening out the most freque
intensity values of the image instead of coefficients. Hence, this technique
known as the histogram equalization. To detect the CLD, unsupervise
learning machine and histogram equalization based feature extraction hav
been developed in the third contribution where it extracts image features a
contrast technique. The basic idea of this mechanism is to find out the enti
affected portion of the image taken from the ultrasound features. Using th
proposed mechanism, only the image features can improve the quality o
image using image enhancement technique. After that segmentation process
done in which the interested area from the background of the image
segmented using k means clustering algorithm. Finally, Haar wavel
decomposition is used to classify the different stages of CLD. Th
experimental outcomes from each phase have proved that all the propose
methods are effective and enhanced the detection and classification fo
solving difficult issues in computer aided diagnosis. Thus, it can be conclude
that the developed proposed mechanisms have met all the research objectiv
stated in chapter 1.

6.1   FUTURE DIRECTIVES

The following are future research directions of the propose
detection and classification mechanisms:

- Mitigating the detected information or disseminatio
  effectiveness is not so much satisfactory because, prior to th
  fast spreading of diseases, and the asymptomatic phenomen
  and negligence of the patients, they may fall under critical stag
  with the considerable changes. Hence, an earlier detectio
  mechanism should be developed for observing the chronic live
  disease.

- Due to complexity, the implementation of the proposed mechanism is not handled correctly in practical situations. So, in the future scope, a smaller mechanism should be developed to overcome practical issues.

- A deep learning method, such as a convolutional network, should be developed to detect and classify the different stages of CLD.